HEALING FOODS

Use the Power of Food to Restore
Your Health, Happiness & Well-Being

Naya Lizardo

Legal Disclaimer

The information provided in this book is designed to provide helpful information regarding the subjects discussed. While best efforts have been used in preparing this book, the author makes no representations or warranties of any kind and assumes no liabilities of any kind with respect to the accuracy or completeness of the contents. The author is not responsible for any specific health or allergy needs that may require medical supervision and is not liable for any damages or negative consequences from any treatment, action, application or preparation, to any person reading or following the information in this book.

Although the foods in this book do contain many health and medicinal properties, they should not be used as a substitute for any medications prescribed to you by your doctor or as a replacement for a doctor's care. You should talk to your doctor before starting any course of therapy or any other treatment.

Printed in the United States of America

First Printing, 2013

ISBN-13: 978-1482636208

ISBN-10: 1482636204

TABLE OF CONTENTS

GASTRO – Bananas

Liver.
Garlic
artichokes
Broccoli
apples.

EYES
Blueberries
Toms

Hair
Spinach

Depression
Beets
Cacao
(raw choc)

Anxiety
Peanuts

anti-inflam
Blueberry
olive oil.
apples – Gout
avacado

Sleep.
Cherry's
spinach
Tuna

warm milk.

INTRODUCTION

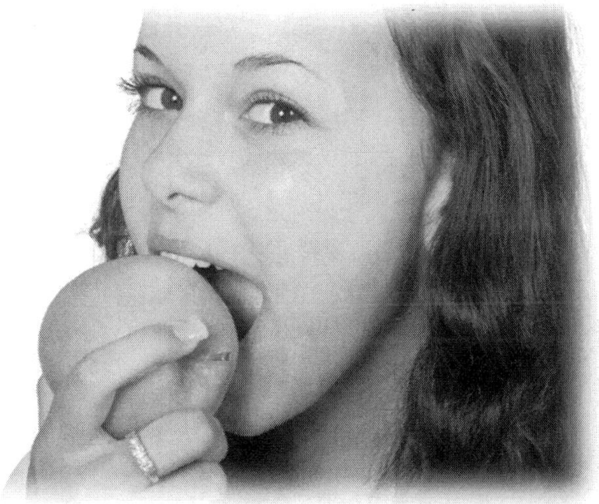

Let your food be your medicine and your medicine be your food.
—Hippocrates

Are you suffering from high cholesterol, diabetes, depression or some other chronic condition? If so, this book may just change your life. Many health conditions can be effectively treated with healing foods.

It's almost impossible to read a magazine or news article without coming across an ad for one pharmaceutical drug or another. These drugs are generally very expensive, but the reader is assured that they are worth ten times the price on account of their wonderful properties and ability to treat or cure everything from acid reflux to high cholesterol to restless leg syndrome. The pharmaceutical companies selling these medications seemingly flourish like flowers in May and spend many thousands of dollars per year in advertising. Many of us are led blindly into wasting our money and often further injuring our health by buying and swallowing drugs about whose properties and effects we know absolutely nothing. But are there alternatives to these pharmaceutical concoctions? Of course there are! Studies are constantly proving that what we eat can often be as or more effective than a prescribed drug. You can use everyday food items to treat everything from high cholesterol to erectile dysfunction.

Vibrant, nutritionally dense foods possess tremendous healing potential. The foods covered in this book are powerful enough to put you in a better mood, help you lower your cholesterol, and reduce your risk of heart disease and cancer. A healthy diet incorporating a variety of these foods will help you prevent and fight disease, as well as maintain your weight, feel younger and live longer.

What is in this book? This book explains what foods can help you prevent and heal a wide variety of ailments and health complaints. Although this book is about using the power of food to address specific health conditions, the book begins by exploring general nutrition and which foods will lead you to better general health. The main part of the book, Part II, focuses on exploring more deeply the health benefits and medicinal uses of particular foods. The last section of this book is organized by health conditions and is intended to serve as a cross reference to the information provided in earlier sections. Filled with science based information, this easy to understand guide will help you reclaim your health, happiness, and well-being.

PART I: Health and Nutrition

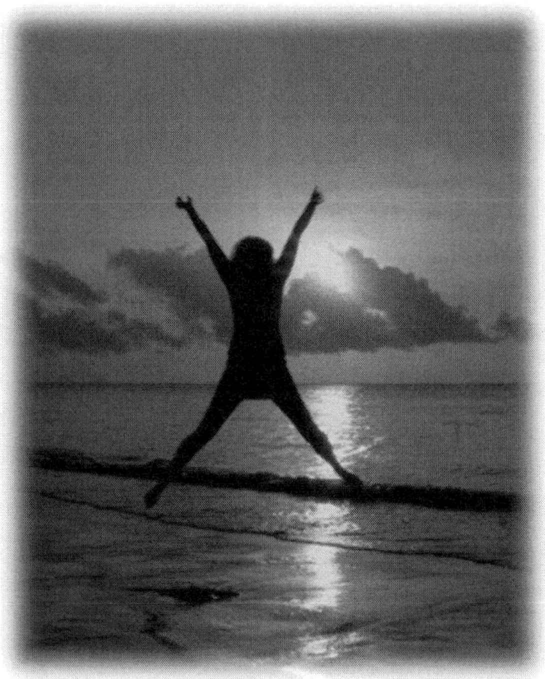

Take care of your body. It's the only place you have to live.
— Jim Rohn

Regaining your health and vitality starts with changing the way you eat. We will begin our path by outlining nutrition basics and exploring foods which will lead you to better overall health.

NUTRITION BASICS

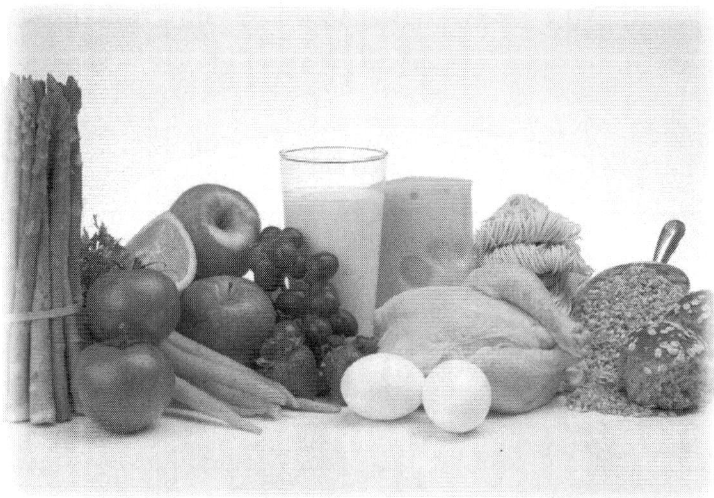

Man Is What He Eats
— Lucretius

Having proper nutrition means that your diet is supplying all the essential nutrients needed by your body to carry out normal tissue growth and repair. If your body has a deficiency in any nutrient it can lead to serious health problems.

The basic components of a healthy diet include the right kinds of proteins, fats, carbohydrates, vitamins and minerals.

Carbohydrates

Carbohydrates provide the body with the fuel it needs for physical activity and for proper organ function. Carbohydrates help regulate fat and metabolize protein. Complex carbohydrates such as whole grains, fruits, vegetables and legumes are the healthiest source of carbohydrates. Complex carbohydrates contain fiber which is important because it decreases the risk for cardiovascular disease and cancer. Simple, easily digested carbohydrates, such white bread, white rice, pastries, sodas, and other highly processed foods, contribute to weight gain and poor health.

Adding Good Carbs to Your Diet

- Eat whole grains hot cereals such as steel cut oats, or low-sugar cold cereals that list a whole grain first on the ingredient list.
- Instead of potatoes, try serving brown rice, bulgur, whole wheat pasta, or another whole grain with your dinner.
- Eat whole fruit instead of drinking juice. An orange has two times as much fiber and only half the sugar as a 12-ounce glass of orange juice.
- Beans are a great source of slowly digested carbohydrate, as well as a great source of protein.

Fats and Cholesterol

Fats and cholesterol are absolutely necessary for good health. Fats cushion vital organs, are used as stored energy, and serve as an insulator to preserve body heat. Cholesterol is a waxy fat-like substance which is an essential part of cells in the body. Cholesterol is used to make certain hormones and to digest fats. The body uses cholesterol to make estrogen, testosterone, vitamin D, and other vital compounds. Cholesterol is so important to our bodies, that the body can actually make all of the cholesterol it needs (about 1000 mg). Most people, however, get some cholesterol from the foods they eat. Only foods from animals, such as meats, dairy and eggs, have dietary cholesterol; plant based foods do not.

Fat and cholesterol are carried through the bloodstream in protein-covered particles called lipoproteins. Low-density lipoproteins (LDL) carry cholesterol from the liver to the rest of the body. When there is too much LDL cholesterol in the blood, it forms deposits or plaques in the artery walls. This plaque narrows the arteries and limit blood flow; heart attacks and strokes are caused when plaque breaks apart. Because of this, LDL cholesterol is often referred to as "bad" cholesterol.

High-density lipoproteins (HDL) are essentially the opposite of LDL cholesterol. High-density lipoproteins go around the body sweeping up as much cholesterol from the bloodstream and artery walls as they can and ferry it back to the liver. HDL also contains antioxidant molecules that help prevent LDL cholesterol from being changed into unhealthy lipoproteins. This is why HDL cholesterol is often referred to as "good" cholesterol.

Triglycerides make up most of the fat consumed in the diet and in the bloodstream. Although, triglycerides are important for good health, an excess of triglycerides can be unhealthy. When we think about fat stored in our thighs or belly, we're thinking of triglycerides. Triglycerides result from the digestion and breaking down of fats in the foods we consume.

The types of dietary fat consumed determine, to a large extent, the amount of HDL and LDL cholesterol, as well as total cholesterol in the bloodstream. Monounsaturated and polyunsaturated fats lower disease risk. Saturated and trans fats increase the risk for disease. Foods high in "good" fats include vegetable oils, nuts, seeds, and fish. Foods high in "bad" fats include red meat, butter, cheese, ice cream, and foods made with partially hydrogenated oil.

Although fat is necessary for our bodies to function, too much fat (especially "bad" fat) can be detrimental to our health (and waistlines). Fats are the most concentrated source of energy; a gram of fat supplies 9 calories to the body. The key to a healthy diet is to choose foods that have more good fats than bad fats; choose vegetable oils instead of butter, salmon instead of steak and choose foods that don't contain any trans fat.

Adding Healthy Fats to Your Diet

- Use liquid plant oils for cooking. Olive oil and other plant-based oils are rich in heart-healthy unsaturated fats.
- Steer clear of trans fat. When purchasing prepackaged products, be sure to read the label to find foods that are free of trans fat. The ingredient list should not contain partially hydrogenated oils. Generally you want to stay away from fried foods, biscuits, and other baked goods.
- Eat at least one good source of omega-3 fatty acids every day. Incorporate fatty fish such as salmon and tuna, walnuts, and olive oil in your diet.
- Eat less milk products and red meat. Red meat and dairy products are high in saturated fat. Get your protein from fish, chicken, nuts, or beans instead. If you eat red meat, be sure to choose lean cuts and keep the portions small.

Proteins

Proteins make up part of every cell, tissue, and organ in our bodies. The protein in the foods we eat is digested and broken down into amino acids that are then used to build and repair tissues including muscles, organs, hair, nails, and bones. Proteins can also be used as a source of energy, but only if the body lacks enough carbohydrates. There are 20 different amino acids that join together to make different types of protein. Our bodies are able to produce some, but not all of these amino acids; these are known as *essential* amino acids.

Complete proteins provide all the essential amino acids needed to build new proteins. Animal sources of protein such as meat, fish and dairy, are generally considered complete proteins. An incomplete protein source is low or lacking in one or more of the essential amino acids. Beans, nuts, and whole grains, are excellent sources of proteins and they offer healthy fiber, vitamins, and minerals, however, they are incomplete proteins. To ensure you get all the amino acids needed to keep your body's systems functioning properly, eat a variety of protein-containing foods each day.

The best animal protein choices are fish and poultry. Clinical research suggests that people who eat red meat have a higher risk of developing heart disease and colon cancer. Eating fish, poultry, beans, or nuts, instead of red meat can help reduce the risk of heart disease and diabetes, and lower the risk of early death.

Include Healthy Proteins in Your Diet:

- Choose lean meats and trim away any fat you can see. For chicken and turkey, be sure to remove the skin.
- Substitute beans for meat in chili and tacos.
- Eat low-fat or fat-free milk, cheese and yogurt.

Vitamins and Minerals

Vitamins and minerals are nutrients that your body needs to grow and function normally. Vitamins and minerals play a unique role in maintaining health. Vitamin D, for example, helps the body absorb the amount of calcium it needs to develop strong bones. Minerals serve several important functions as well. Our bodies use minerals for many different functions, including building bones, making hormones and regulating heartbeat. They are also crucial in maintaining water balance.

Vitamins are classified into two types: fat-soluble (A, D, E, & K) and water-soluble (B complex and C). The body cannot manufacture essential vitamins so they must be obtained through a well-balanced diet.

Fat-Soluble Vitamins

Vitamin A is essential for proper immune function, reproduction, and cellular communication. Vitamin plays a critical role in the normal formation and maintenance of the heart, lungs, kidneys, and other organs. It is also critical for vision because it helps absorb light in the retinal receptors and supports the normal differentiation and functioning of the conjunctival membranes and cornea. Vitamin A can be found both in dark green and yellow fruits and vegetables.

Vitamin D is a fat-soluble vitamin that is naturally present in very few foods. It is manufactured by the body when direct sunlight strikes the skin. Vitamin D promotes calcium absorption and maintains adequate serum calcium and phosphate concentrations. Together with calcium, vitamin D also helps protect older adults from osteoporosis.

Vitamin E is found in a wide variety of foods. Vitamin E is a fat-soluble antioxidant that stops the production of ROS (reactive oxygen species) formed when fat undergoes oxidation. It protects cells from the damaging effects of free radicals therefore helping to prevent or delay chronic diseases associated with free radicals.

Vitamin K is a fat-soluble vitamin that is stored in fat tissue in the liver. It helps blood to clot or coagulate properly. Without it, our blood would not clot. The "K" comes from its German name "Koagulationsvitamin." Vitamin K also plays an important role in bone health. It is produced in the body by bacteria that live in the intestinal tract. Green leafy vegetables like spinach, kale, cabbage, and cauliflower also contain Vitamin K.

Water-Soluble Vitamins

B Vitamins are a group of water-soluble vitamins that play important roles in cell metabolism as well as in maintaining healthy skin and a well-functioning nervous system. The vitamin group includes B1 (thiamine), B2 (riboflavin), B3 (niacin), B5 (pantothenic acid), B6, B7 (biotin), B12 and Folic acid. B vitamins are essential for growth, development, and a variety of other bodily functions. B Vitamins also play a major role in the activities of proteins that regulate chemical reactions in the body, which are important in turning carbohydrates into energy.

Vitamin C is a water-soluble vitamin that is essential for healthy teeth, gums, and blood vessels and for normal growth and development. It helps build the connective tissue that holds body cells together. Vitamin C also helps the body to absorb iron. Because the body cannot make Vitamin C on its own, and it is not stored in the body for long periods of time, it is important to include plenty of vitamin C containing foods in your diet.

Minerals

Like vitamins, minerals help your body grow, develop, and function properly. Minerals help our bodies perform many different functions including building strong bones, transmitting nerve impulses, making hormones, and maintaining a normal heartbeat.

Macrominerals are minerals your body needs in larger amounts. They include calcium, phosphorus, magnesium, sodium, potassium, chloride and sulfur. Trace minerals are only needed in small amounts. These include iron, manganese, copper, iodine, zinc, cobalt, fluoride and selenium.

Calcium is the most abundant mineral in our bodies. Calcium is necessary for critical metabolic functions including vascular contraction and vasodilation, muscle function, nerve transmission, intracellular signaling and hormonal secretion. The rest of the calcium in the body is stored in our bones and teeth, where it supports their structure and function. Dairy products are rich natural sources of calcium. Nondairy sources include vegetables such as kale and broccoli.

Chromium is a trace mineral required by the body in small amounts. Chromium helps enhance the action of insulin, a hormone critical to the metabolism and storage of carbohydrate, fat, and protein in the body.

Iron is required for normal human physiology. It is an essential component of proteins involved in oxygen transport and is also essential for the regulation of cell growth and differentiation. A deficiency of iron will limit the delivery of oxygen to the cells, resulting in fatigue, poor concentration, and decreased immunity. On the other hand, excess of iron can result in toxicity or even death.

Magnesium is essential to good health and is needed for more than 300 biochemical reactions in the body. Magnesium keeps the heart rhythm steady, helps maintain normal muscle and nerve function, supports a healthy immune system, and keeps bones strong. Eating a variety of green leafy vegetables, legumes, nuts, whole grains will help you meet your daily dietary need for magnesium.

Selenium is a trace mineral that is required in small amounts by the body. Selenium has antioxidant properties which help prevent cellular damage from free radicals. Selenium also helps regulate thyroid function and plays a role in the immune system.

Getting the Vitamins and Minerals Your Body Needs:

- The best way to get the vitamins and minerals your body needs is by eating a wide variety of foods. You can usually get all your vitamins from the foods you eat.

EATING FOR OVERALL HEALTH

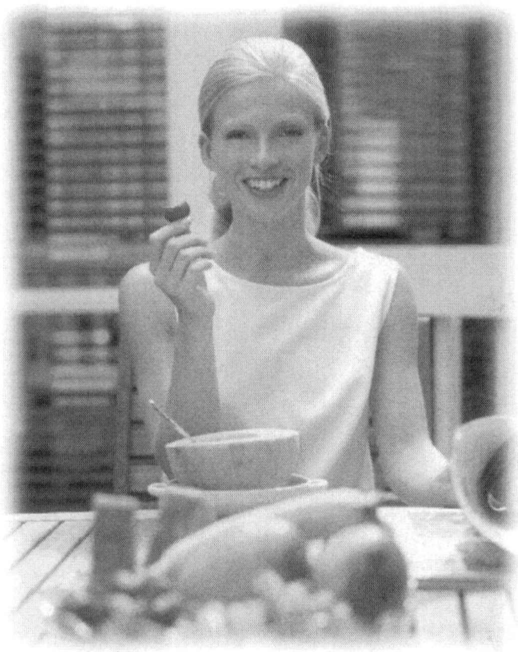

Good food is wise medicine.
—Alison Levitt M.D

What we choose to eat directly affects our feelings of well-being and vitality. Our food choices greatly impact both our physical and mental health and this is true for all of us, despite of our age or current health. Healthy eating is not about staying super thin or depriving yourself of the foods you love; it is about eating foods that bring you health, give you more energy, stabilize your mood and make you feel great.

Trying to switch to a healthy diet overnight isn't realistic or smart. You should begin by taking small, manageable steps. Focus on finding foods you love and easy recipes that incorporate a variety of fresh colorful ingredients. Every change you make to improve your diet is a good change.

Brain Health

The brain is one of the most metabolically active parts of the body and a steady stream of nutrients is needed to fuel the brain. Study after study has found a strong relationship between what we eat and how well we can perform important thinking and memory tasks. Certain nutrients can positively affect the brain, specifically in areas of the brain related to cognitive processing or feelings and emotions. Eating the right foods for our brain not only allows it to function properly but also reduces the risk for cognitive decline.

Avocados

Avocados are excellent in promoting brain health. Avocados lower blood pressure which is a risk factor for the decline in cognitive abilities. They contain monounsaturated fat which contributes to healthy blood flow to the brain.

Blueberries

Blueberries have been called "Brain berries" for a reason. Researchers have found that blueberries help protect the brain from oxidative stress and help reduce the effects of conditions such as Alzheimer's disease or dementia. Diets rich in blueberries have also been shown to improve learning capacity and motor skills.

Eggs

Eggs are rich in choline which is a building block for acetylcholine, a crucial neurotransmitter that is responsible for proper mental functioning. In addition, the cholesterol in eggs has also been found to be beneficial to brain health. Cholesterol supports the membranes of neurons, helping them to keep their shape, and serves as a building block for hormones that influence brain function.

Fatty Fish

Fatty fish like salmon and tuna are rich in Omega-3 fatty acids which are very beneficial for brain health. Omega-3 fatty acids protect the brain and support its development and functioning. In addition, fish is a good source of high quality protein which is important for making the neurotransmitters that improve mental performance.

Sesame Seeds

Sesame seeds are high in zinc which is an important mineral for learning, memory, and brain development. A deficiency in zinc has been linked to cognitive decline. Zinc is also part of the brain's defense system because it promotes immune health and drives enzymes that keep a healthy balance of trace metals in the brain.

Walnuts

There might be a good reason why walnuts look like miniature brains; they are the ultimate brain food. Studies have found that eating walnuts can result in improved cognitive function. The human brain needs high-quality fats like Omega-3's to function properly by keeping the brain fluid and flexible. Walnuts are loaded with Omega-3 fatty acids.

Brain Healthy Appetizer

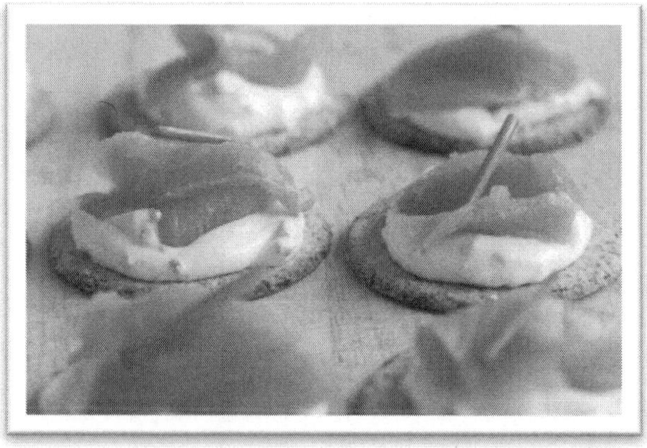

Smoked Salmon Canapés

6 whole wheat crackers
3 tablespoons of sour cream
½ pound of smoked salmon, thinly sliced
1 tablespoon of fresh dills
Freshly ground white pepper
Sea salt
Scallions for Garnish

Mix sourcream and dill. Spread each craker with a little sour cream. Fit salmon slices neatly on top of cracker and achieve some height. Garnish with scallions. Season with pepper and sea salt.

Bone Health

Calcium and vitamin D are key nutrients for building strong healthy bones. Calcium works to build your bones and teeth structure, while vitamin D improves calcium absorption. If you do not consume enough calcium, your body will take the calcium it needs from your bones which could eventually lead to osteoporosis. The best way to get sufficient calcium is to eat enough calcium-rich foods every day.

Dairy Products

It is of course no secret that milk and other dairy products are some of the best sources of calcium and vitamin D, both of which are needed for healthy bones. If you can't consume dairy products due to lactose intolerance or food allergies, there are other good sources of calcium such as tofu, calcium fortified juices and soy milk.

Eggs

Eggs are one of the few whole foods that naturally contain vitamin D, a nutrient that is important in maintaining optimal bone health. They are also an excellent source of nutrients such as calcium, magnesium and vitamins A, which also support bone health.

Fatty Fish

Salmon and tuna are known for having plenty of heart-healthy omega-3 fatty acids, but fatty fish is also great for your bones. A 3-ounce piece of salmon contains more than 100% of your vitamin D. Tuna is also a great source of vitamin D.

Green Leafy Vegetables

Green leafy vegetables are high in vitamin K which is critical in forming bone proteins and reducing calcium loss. Vitamin K has been shown to not only increase bone density in people with osteoporosis, but also reduce fracture rates. One cup of cooked collard greens contains more than 25% of your daily calcium.

Pumpkin Seeds

Magnesium and calcium work together to promote bone health. 50% of the body's magnesium resides in the bones and low levels have been linked to fragile bones. Pumpkin seeds are an excellent source of magnesium.

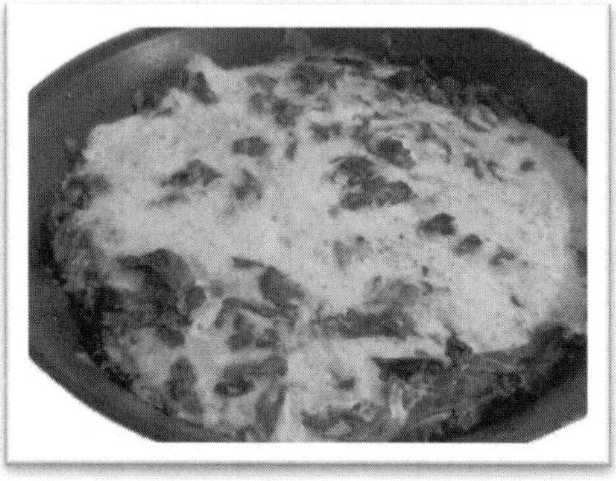

Collard Greens Frittata

1 tablespoon olive oil
1 small yellow onion, chopped
2 cloves garlic, chopped
4 large eggs, beaten
Half a bunch of collard greens, chopped
Salt and Pepper to taste

Preheat oven to 350. Heat oil in 10-inch oven-safe skillet over medium-high heat. Add onion and garlic, and sauté 5 minutes. Add collard greens and season with salt and pepper, and cook until wilted. Pour whisked eggs into skillet. If necessary, tilt the skillet to distribute the eggs and cover the greens. Cook about 3 more minutes or until eggs are almost set but still runny on top. Transfer pan to oven, and bake 14 minutes or until eggs are set. Cut into wedges and serve.

Heart Health

The relationship between diet and heart health has been studied intensively. Every bite of heart-healthy foods delivers a powerful dose of phytonutrients that prevent and repair damage to cells and help prevent heart disease.

Fruits and Vegetables

Fruits and vegetables are high in antioxidants, folate, fiber, and potassium. These nutrients blunt the effects of free radical damage to the heart and help prevent heart disease. Eating a diet rich in fruits and vegetables is linked with a lower risk of heart attacks, strokes, heart failure and death from heart disease.

Oatmeal

Oatmeal is high in B-vitamins which are effective in lowering homocycsteine levels associated with cardiovascular diseases. Oatmeal is also high in a specific type of fiber called beta-glucans which helps protect the heart and lowers LDL cholesterol. People with high cholesterol who consume one bowl of oatmeal a day typically lower their total cholesterol by 8-20%.

Dark Chocolate!

Chocolate is high in flavonoids which help protect the cardiovascular system and inhibit platelet clumping. Research indicates that the flavonoids in chocolate reduce cell damage associated with heart disease, lower blood pressure, and improve vascular function.

Olive Oil

The main type of fat found in olive oil is monounsaturated fatty acids. Monounsaturated fats have been shown to reduce the inflammation often associated with the risk for cardiovascular disease. Olive oil helps to lower your total cholesterol and low-density lipoprotein cholesterol levels.

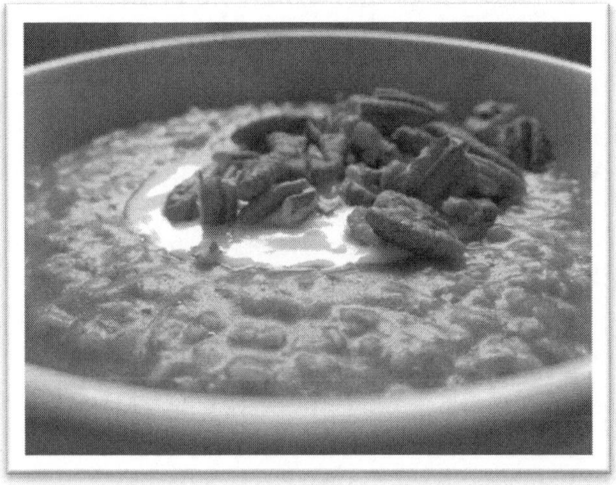

Pumpkin Spice Oatmeal

1 cup old-fashioned oats
1/2 cup pureed canned pumpkin
1 cup skim milk
1 teaspoon of cinnamon
Dash of ground cloves
Dash of ground nutmeg
Handful of pecans (optional)

Put the oats and milk into a small pot on the stove. Stir continuously over medium high heat until the mixture gets thick and creamy (about 5 minutes). Reduce heat to medium low and add the canned pumpkin and the spices. Top with pecans.

Healthy Aging

You already know that eating nutritious foods can help you stay healthy, but what you eat can also make a difference on how you age, from the inside out. Making wise decisions about what you eat as you get older is very important. Aging can take a toll on many parts of our bodies including eyes, bones, skin, heart, and mind.

Fatty Fish

Omega-3 fatty acids commonly found in fish oils offer many anti-aging benefits. Omega-3 fatty acids are considered essential fatty acids and are vital for normal metabolism. They protect your heart and reduce your risk of stroke. Studies also suggest that consuming omega-3 fatty acids can reduce the risk of age related dementia.

Brazil Nut

Constipation is common at all ages, but as we age we tend to be more susceptible. Adding brazil nuts to your diet may provide much needed relief. Brazil nuts are high in selenium and fiber which help get things moving.

Fruits and Vegetables

Fruits and vegetables provide fiber, vitamins, and minerals and many other anti-aging phytonutrients. These phytonutrients will help to boost your energy, ward off the signs of aging and may even reverse age-related brain decline. When it comes to fighting the effects of aging, fruits and vegetables can really work wonders. They may not be miracle pills, but they can certainly help you live longer. By eating a diet rich in fruits and vegetables, you will not only add years to your life, but you can also look as great as you feel!

Anti-Aging Dinner

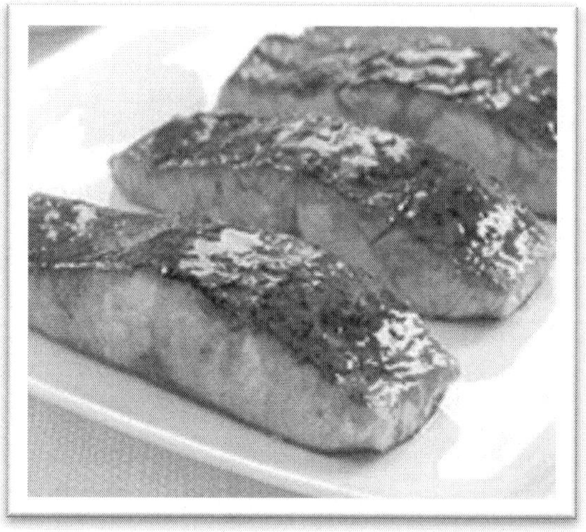

Soy Glazed Salmon

4 tablespoons of olive oil
2 tablespoons soy sauce
1 tablespoons of lemon juice
2 tablespoons of water
1 ½ pounds of salmon fillet

Preheat oven to 400 degrees. In a small bowl, mix together the olive oil, soy sauce, lemon juice, and water. Cut salmon fillet into 4 equal-size pieces and arrange, skin side down, in a single layer in a baking dish. Pour glaze over the fish coating evenly. Bake 15 minutes or until fish is opaque but still bright pink inside, basting every few minutes with glaze from baking dish.

Healthy Skin

The secret to a beautiful, wrinkle-free complexion lies in what you eat. Eating the right foods can help you fight acne, minimize wrinkles, and enhance your skin's natural beauty.

Salmon

Salmon has one of the richest concentration omega-3 fatty acids, which help fortify skin cell membranes, protect against sun damage, and reduce the risk of certain forms of skin cancer. These healthy fats allow water and nutrients into the skin, keep toxins out, and reduce the body's production of inflammatory substances, decreasing clogged pores, and averting fine lines and wrinkles.

Sweet Potatoes

The sweet potato's orange flesh color is directly correlated to its beta-carotene content. Sweet potatoes boast large amounts of this valuable nutrient which helps combat rough winter skin and may also help protect against UV damage and wrinkles.

Broccoli

Broccoli is high in antioxidants, including vitamins C and E which aid in the production of collagen, protects your skin cell membranes, guard against UV radiation damage, and keep your skin healthy and supple.

Sunflower Seeds

Sunflower seeds are replete with vitamin E, a powerful antioxidant that slows down the aging of skin cells and diminishes the appearance of scars. These seeds are also high in zinc which helps maintain collagen and promotes skin renewal.

Skin Healthy Soup

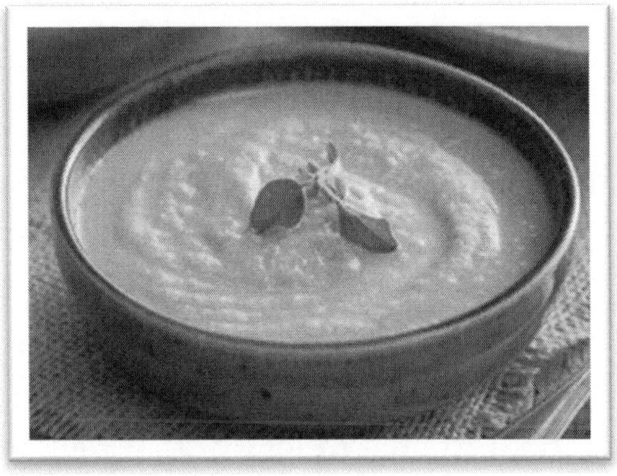

Creamy Sweet Potato Soup

1 tablespoons of olive oil
2 cloves garlic, peeled, chopped
1 ½ cups of chicken stock
2 baked sweet potato, skin removed
Salt and pepper to taste
¼ of cup of heavy cream

Add the olive oil to a sauce pan and saute the garlic for one minute. Add the onion, salt and pepper, and cook for five minutes or until tender, stirring occasionally. Add the chicken stock and sweet potato and bring to a rolling boil, stirring to combine. Reduce heat, add cream and simmer for eight minutes. Remove from heat and blend the soup until smooth.

Weight Management

It's no secret that the foods you eat are directly linked to your weight. The results of a study recently published in *The New England Journal of Medicine* showed that small changes in lifestyle behaviors such as physical activity and sleep duration are strongly correlated with long-term weight gain; however the most important factor was food.

There are of course foods that promote weight gain and foods that promote weight loss. We all know the common culprits that drive weight gain (fried foods, sugar, sweetened beverages, processed meats, and starchy carbs) but here are some of the best foods to help you lose or maintain your weight.

Vegetables

Daily intake of vegetables can help speed up your weight loss because they are low in calories, high in volume, and packed with nutrients and fiber. In essence, they fill you up without all the calories, thus controlling cravings and overeating.

Citrus Fruits and Berries:

Fruits in general are an excellent source of energy and nutrition. Diets rich in fruits provide the required nutrients to the body and keep the body hydrated. Citrus fruits and berries are low in carbohydrates. A diet rich in citrus fruits and berries can be a good way to detoxify the body and help with weight loss. These fruits aid in removing bad cholesterol, improving digestion and decreasing appetite, thereby leading to healthy weight loss.

Whole Grains

Whole grains are naturally low-fat and cholesterol free. They also and contain fiber, which helps curb your appetite. Because of their fiber content, whole grains are low in the glycemic index which means that they are absorbed into your bloodstream slowly, allowing you to go longer without feeling those hunger pangs or cravings.

Yogurt

Adding yogurt to your diet helps you lose weight by increasing your body's ability to burn fat, especially that stubborn belly fat. Your stored belly fat produces the hormone cortisol, which signals your body to store more body fat. The calcium in yogurt helps break this cycle by signaling your fat cells to produce less cortisol. The amino acids in yogurt also help you burn calories. According to a study published in the *International Journal of Obesity,* obese adults who ate three servings of fat-free yogurt daily as part of a lower-calorie diet lost 22% more weight and 61% more body fat than those who just cut calories. In addition, yogurt eaters also lost 81% more belly fat.

Nuts

Nuts are good sources of protein and fiber and contain many essential vitamins your body needs. Nuts are also full of healthy fats, which create a feeling of satiety. The more satisfied you feel, the less you are likely to snack excessively between meals or overeat during the meals. While nuts do have a large amount of calories and fat, if you eat them in controlled portions they will be very beneficial for your weight loss efforts. Research has shown that people who eat nuts lose more weight, so don't be afraid to include them in your weight loss plan.

Diet Friendly Dinner

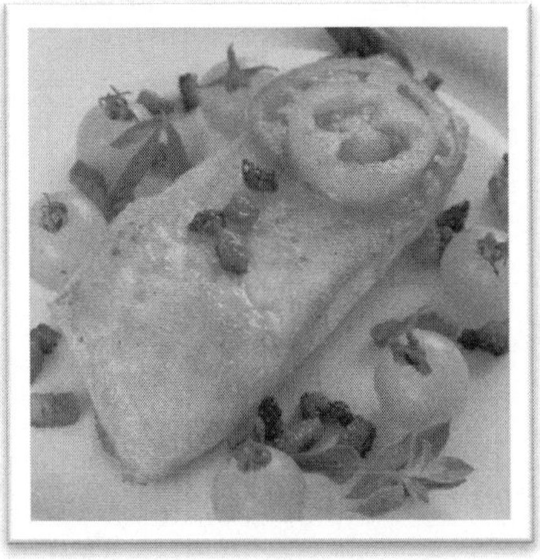

Roasted Fish with Cherry Tomatoes

1 pound white fleshed fish
1 cup cherry tomatoes
2 teaspoons extra-virgin olive oil
5 garlic cloves, peeled
Salt and pepper to taste

Preheat oven to 425 degrees. In a baking pan, combine tomatoes, oil, garlic, salt and pepper. Roast for 15 minutes. Remove from oven. Place fish in pan with tomatoes. Continue roasting 10 more minutes or until fish is no longer translucent.

PART II: Food Cures

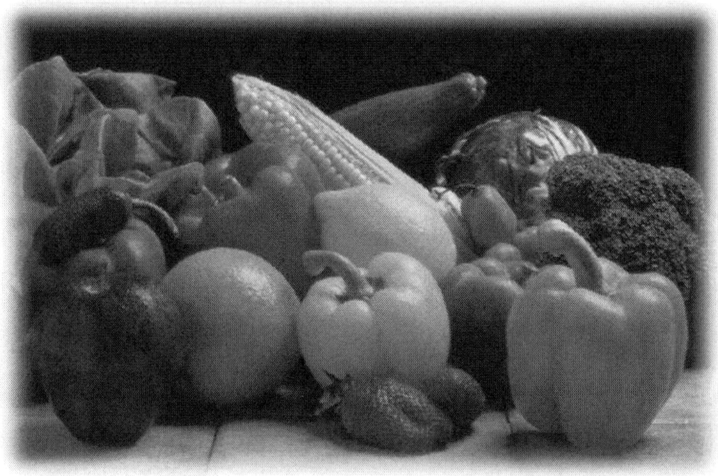

The doctor of the future will no longer treat the human frame with drugs, but rather will cure and prevent disease with nutrition.
—Thomas Edison

Using food as medicine is nothing new, but it is too often overlooked as a real and effective solution to many health problems. Many people are also unaware of the specific medicinal uses and health benefits of particular foods. This section is dedicated to exploring this further. Here we will look at the healing powers of variety of power foods.

FRUITS

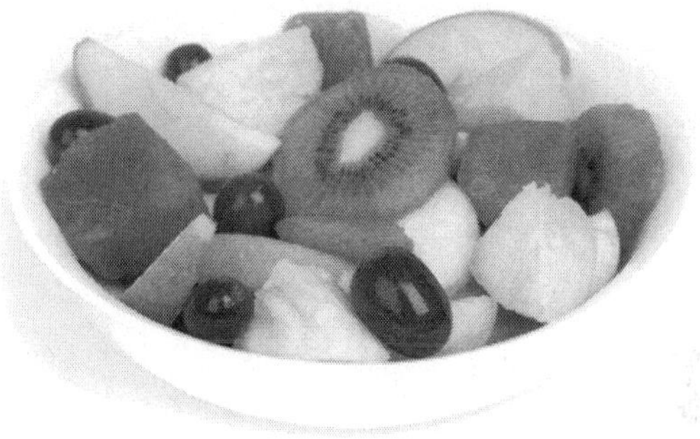

A table, a chair, a bowl of fruit and a violin; what else does a man need to be happy.
—Albert Einstein

Fruits are nature's amazing medicines packed with vitamins, minerals, antioxidants and many phytonutrients. Antioxidants help protect the human body from oxidative stress, diseases, and cancers, as well as boost our immunity level. Fruits are also a good source of soluble fiber, which helps to lower cholesterol and provide relief from constipation. Vitamins and minerals are found in most foods, but fruits are particularly good sources of many of these valuable compounds.

Apples

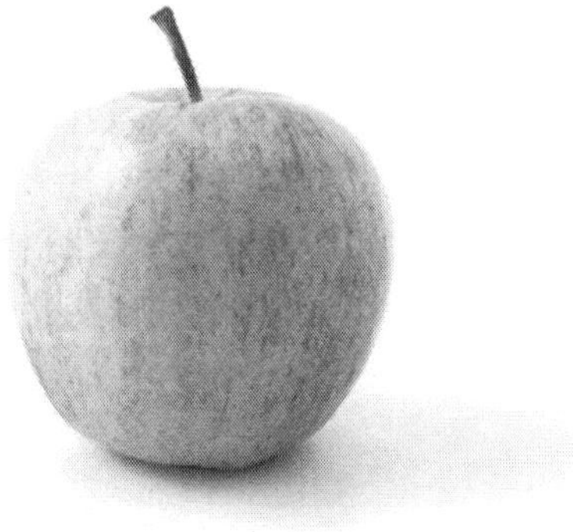

Apples have surprising nutritional benefits that justify the old "apple a day" adage. The apple has definitely earned its place as a symbol of health. The majority of the health benefits come from its phosphorus content and its more than 250 phytochemicals.

Alzheimer's Disease

Eating apples can improve your memory and help you sustain overall brain health. Apples contain a larger percentage of phosphorus than any other fruit or vegetable. For this reason it is an invaluable food for brain health. The effects of the antioxidants and flavonoids present in apples have been shown to reduce brain-cell inflammation and oxidation that occurs naturally due to the presence of free radicals. Eating apples increases acetylcholine, which is a critical neurotransmitter for memory and brain health. Eating apples has been shown to diminish accumulations of toxins in the brain, particularly beta-amyloid, which is thought to be one of the main factors causing Alzheimer's Disease.

Gout

Gout occurs when the body has high levels of uric acid and is characterized by recurrent attacks of acute inflammatory arthritis. Gout symptoms occur when excess uric acid forms sharp crystals which collect between the joints and cause painful inflammation. The malic acid contained in apples helps to neutralize uric acid. Daily consumption of apples can help reduce gout attacks.

Heart Disease

Apples are full of antioxidant compounds which help inhibit inflammation and lower levels of cholesterol and two other markers associated with plaque and inflammation in artery walls. Apples are also high in fiber which has been shown to lower cholesterol level. Studies have shown that frequent apple eaters have reduced risk of suffering from heart attacks and strokes compared with non-apple eaters.

Liver Ailments

Your liver plays a vital role in your health and vitality. Having a healthy liver results in greater energy and general sense of well-being. A poorly functioning liver can result in tiredness, headaches, allergies, problem skin, and weight gain. Apples periodically appear on the dinner table in the form of apple sauce or chutneys to accompany dishes like roast pork or pork chops for a reason. The cook who created this menu was evidently acquainted with the action of the fruit on the liver. Apples contain pectin which keeps the liver from absorbing cholesterol and binds to heavy metals in the body (in particular in the colon) to help their excretion. This reduces the load on the liver and its detoxification capacities. The malic acid in apples also helps to break up gall stones.

Parkinson's Disease

Parkinson's disease is a disorder of the nervous system that develops gradually and affects movement. Parkinson's disease cannot be cured; however apples could help to decrease the onset of

Parkinson's. Researchers at Harvard University found that the flavonoids in apples help stave off Parkinson's in men.

Weight Loss

Apples can be part of a healthy diet that promotes weight loss because they satisfy hunger with only a few calories. A study at Florida State University showed that eating a cup of dried apples daily can help women lose weight and lower their cholesterol and heart disease markers. In addition, according to the *National Health and Nutrition Examination Survey,* diets high in dried fruits are associated with lower Body Mass Index (BMI) and improved diet quality.

Avocado

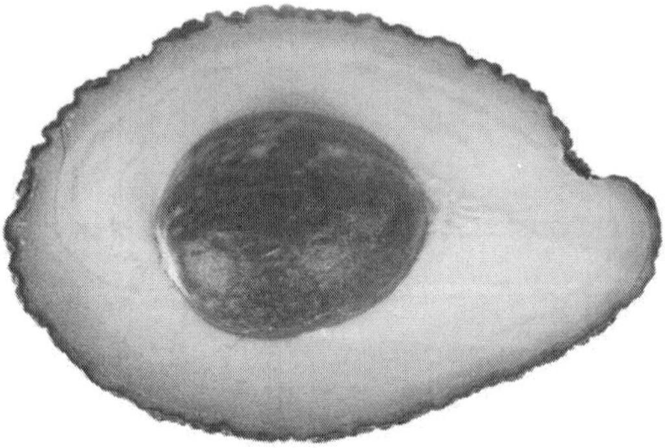

Avocados are an amazing superfood with a rich flavor and powerful wide-ranging health benefits. Among other benefits, avocados improve cardiovascular health, stabilize blood sugar, and reduce cholesterol. Avocados are rich in folate, potassium, vitamin E, magnesium, fiber, and heart healthy monounsaturated fats. Avocados contain more folate per ounce than any other fruit, with 90 micrograms per cup. Folate (folic acid) deficiency has been linked to a variety of diseases and conditions including atherosclerosis, heart attacks and strokes, as well as birth defects and congenital abnormalities. For this reason, avocados are one of the healthiest things you can add to your diet.

Heart Disease

Avocados are high in folic acid which has been found to reduce the levels of homocysteine in the blood. Lower levels of homocysteine reduce the risks of heart disease and blood vessel disease. Research suggests that folate deficiencies may trigger up to 40% percent of the heart attacks and strokes suffered by men in the U.S. every year. The risk of heart disease can be greatly reduced by an increased intake of dietary folate. As mentioned above, avocados contain approximately 90 micrograms of folic acid per cup. Avocados are also the only fruit that contains monounsaturated fat, which helps protect against heart disease.

High Cholesterol

Cholesterol lowering foods should be included into everyone's diet. Avocados are one such food. The oleic acid in avocados can help lower total cholesterol and LDL cholesterol levels while increasing the HDL (good cholesterol) levels. Avocados are also rich in fiber and beta-sitosterol, both of which help keep cholesterol levels low.

Inflammation

Avocados have been clinically shown to help reduce inflammation. Avocados contain many anti-inflammatory agents including phytosterols, carotenoid antioxidants and omega-3 fatty acids. They are rich in anti-inflammatory monounsaturated oleic fatty acids that help balance out the often pro-inflammatory polyunsaturated omega-6 fats. Phytosterols also help prevent pro-inflammatory prostaglandin-E2 synthesis by the connective tissue. Inflammation diseases like arthritis respond very well to diets high in phytosterols.

Weight Loss

If eaten moderately, avocados can play a role in weight loss diets. While they are high in calories, their high monounsaturated fat content helps to increase feelings of satiety. In addition, research suggests that exercise burns monounsaturated fat more efficiently than saturated fat.

Bananas

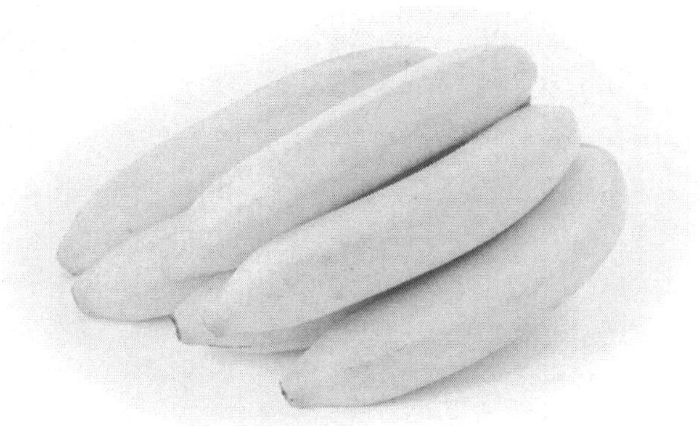

Bananas are commonly considered to be a healthy food. They are a great source of potassium, iron, fiber and other vitamins and have been known to alleviate a number of short and long term conditions.

Anemia

Bananas are high in iron which is essential for the production of hemoglobin, myoglobin, and enzymes essential in the production of red blood cells. They are therefore an excellent food for anemic persons.

Gastrointestinal Problems

Bananas are a good choice to settle an upset digestive system. Bananas normalize colonic functions in the large intestine by absorbing large amounts of water. The high level of potassium in bananas helps to replace electrolytes that may be lost during bouts of diarrhea. Bananas also contain insoluble fiber, which helps relieve constipation. They also contain inulin, a prebiotic soluble fiber that promotes the growth of beneficial bacteria in the intestinal system.

Muscular Cramps

A deficiency in potassium can cause muscle cramps and spasms, as well as greater susceptibility to injury. Bananas are high in potassium and thus can help relieve muscle cramps and spasms.

Blackberries

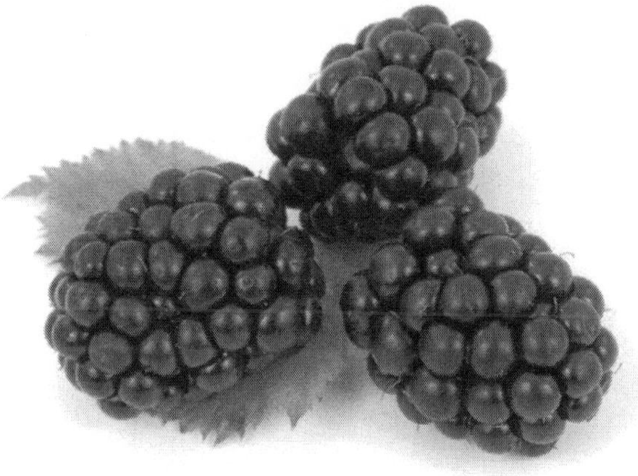

Eating fruits rich in blue pigments such as blueberries and blackberries offers many health benefits. These fruits have potent antioxidant properties which help remove free radicals from the body thus protecting against infections, aging, and even cancer. Blackberries have numerous other health benefits.

Cancer

Blackberries are particularly rich in anthocyanins, which have antioxidant and anti-inflammatory properties. According to a study published *The*

Journal of Biological Chemistry, the anthocyanins in blackberries may help prevent or inhibit the growth of cancerous cells. In addition, the high concentration of antioxidants found in blackberries may help prevent free radical mediated damage, thereby reducing the risk of chronic conditions such as cancer.

Diarrhea

Blackberries are one of the best foods around for the treatment of diarrhea. Blackberries contain tannins that help to tone the intestinal tract and soothe diarrhea. They also help prevent the irritating and toxic substances that cause diarrhea from being absorbed back into the bloodstream.

Heart Disease

Blackberries may help to prevent heart disease by inactivating the enzymes that damage the endothelial cells lining the blood vessels. They contain high amounts of fiber, are rich in polyphenols, vitamin C, and contain a bit of iron, calcium, and vitamin A. The antioxidants in blackberries also protect the cells of the cardiovascular system from harmful effects of unstable oxygen radicals.

Inflammation

Inflammation is really the cause of a lot of our ill health. As we age, we become more susceptible to free radical damage and inflammation. Blackberries are full of antioxidants which protect the body against inflammation and free radicals. More specifically, studies have shown that the phenolic components of blackberries exhibit powerful anti-inflammatory properties and inhibit the activity of inflammatory chemicals such as interleukins.

Blueberries

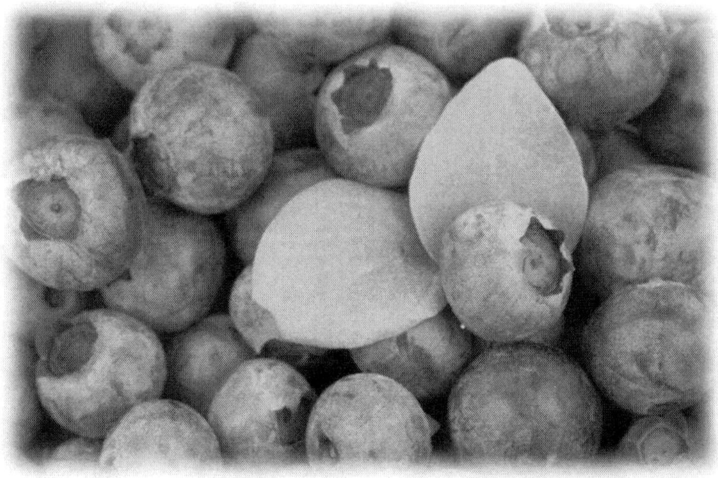

Blueberries have the highest antioxidant capacity of all fresh fruit. They are rich in antioxidants like anthocyanin, vitamin C, B complex, vitamin E, vitamin A, as well as copper, selenium, zinc, and iron.

Cancer

Blueberries contain phenolic compounds which, in harmony with anthocyanin and other antioxidants can do wonders to prevent or treat cancers. Studies published in the *Journal of Agricultural and Food Chemistry* showed that the phenolic compounds in blueberries can inhibit colon cancer cell proliferation. Another study at the Beckman Research Institute showed that blueberries have the potential to inhibit the growth of Triple Negative Breast Cancer, a particularly aggressive form of breast tumor.

Heart Disease

Blueberries have a high anthocyanin content. Anthocyanin has been shown to dilate arteries, counter the buildup of plaque, and provide other cardiovascular benefits. Blueberries are also rich in fiber and antioxidants which help reduce the likelihood of heart attacks. A Harvard School of Public Health study published in the January 2013 issue of the *Journal of the American Heart Association,* found that eating three or more servings of blueberries per week may reduce a woman's risk of heart attack by as much as 33%.

Inflammation

Blueberries are excellent anti-inflammatories and pain relievers. Blueberries increase the amounts of compounds called heat-shock proteins which help reduce inflammation and pain. Blueberries also contain salicylic acid which is the natural version of aspirin and is known to thin the blood and reduce pain.

Memory Problems

When it comes to brain health, there really is nothing quite like blueberries, some have even called them "brain berries." Blueberries are high in anthocyanins which help prevent the breakdown of brain cells. Studies have found that people who eat at least one cup of blueberries per week experience less mental decline compared to those who rarely eat them. In addition to anthocyanin, blueberries contain selenium, vitamins A, B-complex, C, and E, zinc, sodium, potassium, copper, magnesium, phosphorus, and manganese. These power-packed berries can help prevent degeneration and death of neurons and brain-cells and restore health of the central nervous system. Blueberries help protect the brain from oxidative stress and may reduce the effects of age-related memory impairments like dementia and even Alzheimer's. Blueberries have even been shown to improve learning capacity.

Urinary Tract Infections

Everybody knows that cranberries help fight urinary tract infections, but for those of us who do not appreciate their tartness, blueberries are an excellent choice. Blueberries have been shown to be quite beneficial to urinary tract health. Bacteria like b-coli are responsible for urinary tract infections.

Blueberries have a compound which inhibits the growth of these bacteria. Blueberries also have some antibiotic properties which add to this effect.

Vision Problems

Blueberries have the potential to slow down visual loss and prevent or delay age related ocular problems like macular degeneration and cataract due to their high levels of antioxidants. The antioxidant in blueberries include carotenoids (lutein, zeaxanthin), flavonoids (resveritrol, quercetin), vitamin C, vitamins E and A, selenium, zinc and phosphorus, which are very beneficial to ocular health.

Weight Loss

Blueberries contain catechin, which is a natural phenol and antioxidant known to activate fat-burning in abdominal fat cells. Studies have shown that eating blueberries regularly increases abdominal fat loss and total weight loss.

Cherries

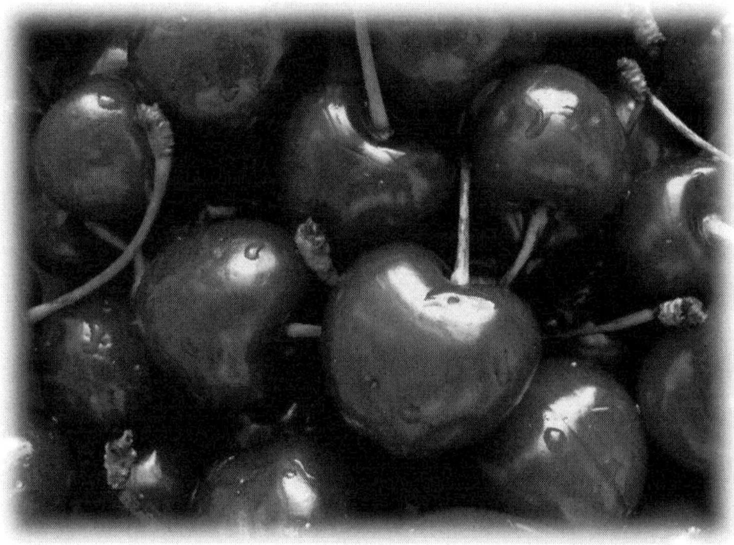

Cherries are not only delicious, but they have many health benefits. Cherries are rich in polyphenolic flavonoid compounds known as anthocyanin glycosides. Cherries have potential health effects against chronic painful episodes such as arthritis, fibromyalgia, and sports injuries.

Muscle Pain

If you're looking for a healthy way to ease post-exercise muscle pain and soreness, cherries might be a great option. Cherries contain the same anti-inflammatory enzymes as Ibuprofen, without the potential side effects. Cherries contain high levels of polyphenols, which reduce inflammation, tenderness and pain.

Sleep Problems

Nothing is worse than insomnia or poor sleep. Not only is it frustrating, but research has shown that poor sleep can be detrimental to our health. The antioxidant melatonin significantly improves the body's sleep pattern and sleep quality. Cherries are one of the few foods that contain melatonin. Cherries can increase melatonin levels in the blood therefore improving the way you sleep. A cup of tart cherries or glass of tart cherry juice can improve the duration and quality of your sleep.

Coconut

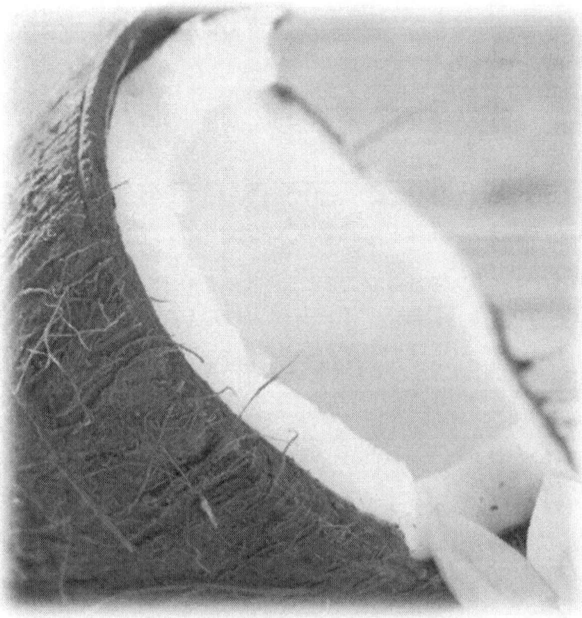

Coconuts contain properties that can be helpful in a wide range of ailments from heart disease to Alzheimer's. Unfortunately, coconut is one of those foods whose health benefits are often hotly argued over. Although some argue that the high levels of saturated fats in coconut make it a less than ideal food, there is a lot of evidence supporting the many health benefits of this mighty fruit. Coconut oil is composed predominately of medium-chain triglycerides (MCTs) which are distinctly different from the long-chain fatty acids more commonly found in unhealthy high-fat diets. It is these MCTs that give coconut many of its healing properties.

Heart Diseases

Many people can't imagine how a food high in saturated fat, like the coconut, can be beneficial for the heart. Extra virgin coconut oil is beneficial for the heart because it contains about 50% lauric acid, which helps in preventing various heart problems including high cholesterol levels and high blood pressure. In addition, the saturated fats present in coconut oil are Medium Chain Triglycerides (MCT's) which do not lead to an increase in LDL levels. The coconut actually protects against heart disease by increasing good cholesterol and lowering the ratio of bad and good cholesterol.

IBS

Extra virgin coconut oil has been shown to help improve the digestive system and thus prevent various stomach and digestion related problems including irritable bowel syndrome. The saturated fats present in coconut oil have antimicrobial properties which can help control the bacteria, fungi and parasites that cause indigestion and irritable bowel symptoms.

Weight Loss

Extra virgin coconut oil can be a helpful tool in your weight loss efforts. It contains short and medium-chain fatty acids that help in taking off excessive weight. Coconut is easy to digest and it helps in healthy functioning of the thyroid and enzymes systems. It also helps to increase body metabolism and energy because it is more likely to be burned as fuel than stored as body fat.

Grapefruit

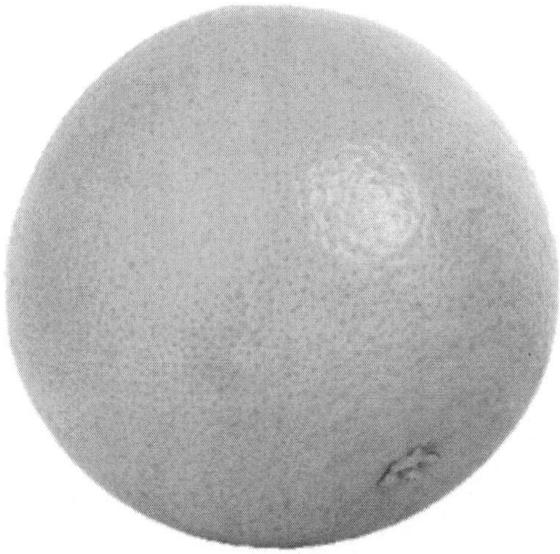

Grapefruits are a great source of vitamin C which has been shown to relieve the severity of cold symptoms and to protect our bodies against oxidative stress. But there's a lot more to grapefruits than vitamin C.

> *Warning: If you are taking any kind of prescription medication, please check with your doctor before adding grapefruit to your diet. There have been known interactions between grapefruit and prescription medications.*

Cancer

Pink and red grapefruits are excellent sources of lycopene. Lycopene has a high capacity to help fight oxygen free radicals and is a powerful agent against tumors and cancers. Grapefruit also contains liminoids and naringenin. Liminoids may help prevent cancerous cells from proliferating and also inhibit tumor formation by promoting the formation of glutathione-S-transferase, a detoxifying enzyme. Naringenin is an antioxidant compound which has been shown to repair damaged DNA in prostate cancer cells.

High-Cholesterol

Grapefruits can help reduce cholesterol levels. Grapefruits are high in antioxidants and contain pectin, a soluble fiber that has been shown to slow down the progression of atherosclerosis. Studies have shown that grapefruits can reduce blood levels of LDL cholesterol and triglycerides. Both red and blond grapefruits can positively influence cholesterol levels, but red grapefruit is more effective, especially in lowering triglycerides.

Weight Loss

Research suggests that the chemical properties of grapefruit reduce insulin levels and encourage weight loss. Grapefruits have high amounts of fat burning enzymes, high water content, fiber and low glycemic load. A combination of these characteristics makes grapefruit a perfect food for losing weight.

Kiwi

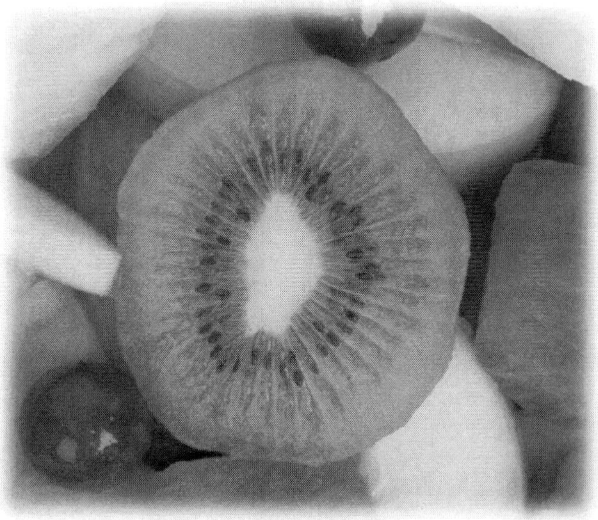

The kiwi offers an array of health-promoting nutrients. Kiwis are rich in vitamin C, and also contain vitamin E, folate, potassium, fiber, carotenoids, polyphenols, chlorophyll, glutathione, and pectin. In fact, kiwis contain more vitamin C than oranges, more fiber than apples and more potassium than bananas.

Heart Disease

Kiwi can be considered a superfood for your heart. The Cleveland Clinic has recommended kiwis as one of the most powerful foods for the heart. Kiwis help to lower triglyceride levels and reduce platelet hyperactivity which plays a role in the development and stability of atherosclerotic vascular plaques and limits the tendency of blood to form clots. The vitamin C and E in kiwis, combined with the polyphenols and magnesium, potassium, B vitamins, and copper, act to protect the cardiovascular system.

Respiratory Problems

Your lungs are constantly bombarded by toxins, such as air pollution, cigarette smoke and allergens. This exposure can lead to lung cancer, bronchitis and other respiratory ailments. This nutrient dense fruit pack more vitamin C than oranges and is especially effective against respiratory problems such as shortness of breath, asthma and cough. Studies indicate that kiwi eaters are less likely to experience wheezing, shortness of breath, or runny noses.

Lemon

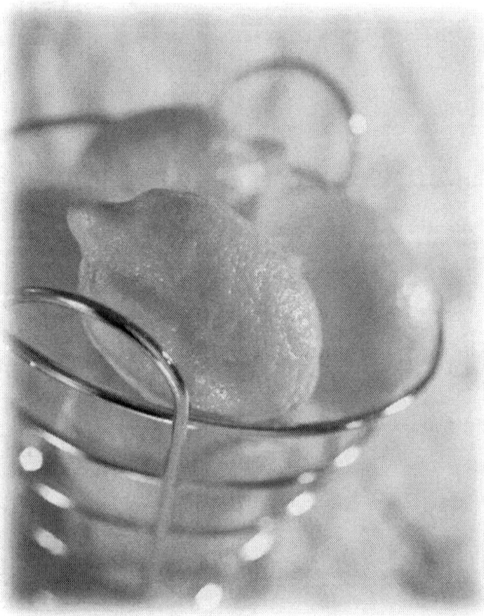

Lemons pack a strong phytochemical punch; they are one of those super foods with a myriad health benefits. Lemons have been used by cultures around the world since ancient times to improve and maintain health. Lemons contain bioflavonoids, which are antioxidant chemicals believed to be responsible for its beneficial health effects.

Acne

Acne occurs when skin cells, sebum, and hair clump together plugging hair follicles which then become infected with bacteria, resulting in a swelling. While your instinct might be to run to the drugstore to purchase acne treatments, you can find an excellent treatment for your acne right in your refrigerator. Lemons have healing properties that work well to heal acne blemishes. Lemon juice can be applied directly to the skin or drunk as a beverage. Applied externally, lemons decrease inflammation, redness and irritation from acne and restore skin to health. Lemons are rich in vitamin C which has anti-inflammatory properties and alpha-hydroxy acid which works as a skin exfoliator. Lemons have disinfectant properties; the acid in lemon juice breaks down the main acne-causing bacteria, p. acnes. Internally, lemons works by stopping signals to the immune system to cause inflammation.

Canker Sores

Canker sores should not be confused with cold sores. Cold sores or fever blisters are caused by a virus and typically appear outside of the mouth. Canker sores, on the other hand, are small ulcers that appear inside of the mouth and can make eating and talking quite uncomfortable. Canker sores may be small, but they can be hard to ignore. Fortunately, a canker sore is are generally pretty short-lived, but lemons can provide some temporary relief. Lemons have antibacterial properties which can accelerate the healing process of canker sores. Mix the juice of freshly squeezed lemon into a glass of lukewarm water and rinse your mouth with this solution several times a day.

Halitosis

Although lemons might be mouth-puckering to the taste, the citric acid in lemons can help to neutralize bad-breath smells. Chewing on fresh lemons or rinsing with lemon juice can help freshen breath after consuming certain foods, spices, alcohol, or cigarettes.

Kidney Stones

If you've ever passed a kidney stone, you won't forget the sudden, intense pain. Kidney stones form when urine in the kidney becomes supersaturated with stone-forming salts. Lemon juice increases the amount of citrate in the urine which helps to inhibit kidney stones from forming. If you are prone to kidney stones, you may want to consider drinking low sugar or sugar-free lemonade on a regular basis. Scientific evidence suggests that drinking 1 to 2 liters of lemon juice as lemonade per day can help you lower the risk of developing kidney stones.

Meniere's disease

Meniere's disease is an idiopathic disease involving the inner ear that is characterized by vertigo, hearing loss and pain, nausea and tinnitus. Meniere's disease does not have a cure; however lemons may bring some relief to those who suffer from this disease. Research has shown that Meniere's disease patients treated with lemon bioflavonoid complex saw improvements in their vertigo and hearing symptoms. Although the exact physiologic mechanism by which this effect is produced is unknown, it is hypothesized that the bioflavonoids in lemon may act as a blocking agent on histidine decarboxylase.

Sore Throat

An inflamed sore throat can be difficult to cope with. Sore throats are often caused by allergies, bacterial infections or viral infections including the common cold. Sore throats are often accompanied by fever, chills, swollen lymph nodes and pain while swallowing. Lemon and honey mixture makes an excellent sore throat relieving alternative.

Honey has been proven effective against many kinds of bacteria and lemons enhance the antimicrobial properties of the honey. Lemons are also high in vitamin C which boosts the immune system. Lemons also work to reduce inflammation and thin mucous congestion.

Mango

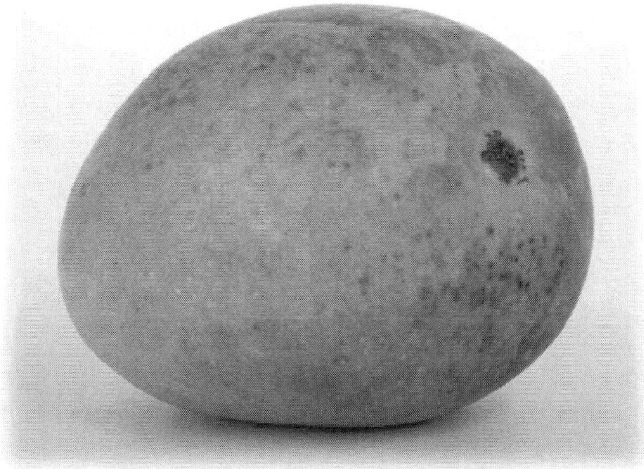

Mangoes taste so delicious that people often forget how healthy they really are. Mangoes are high in vitamin A, vitamin C, vitamins B1 and B2, niacin, potassium, iron, and fiber. They are good for the kidneys, digestive system and the skin.

Acid Reflux

Acid reflux occurs when digestive fluid backs up past the lower esophageal sphincter into your esophagus. When this happens, you feel a burning pain in your chest or abdomen. The tartaric acid, malic acid, and a trace of citric acid found in mangoes help to neutralize acid. The juice of the mango also coats the lining of the esophagus, relieving any pain caused by the acid moving upwards.

Cancer

Mangoes are rich in phenols, such as quercetin, isoquercitrin, astragalin, fisetin, gallic acid and methylgallat, and enzymes which have cancer preventing capacities. Mangoes are also high in a soluble fiber which has been linked to a lower risk of cancers of the gastrointestinal tract. Mangoes also provide vitamin C which helps protect cells from free radical damage and reduces the risk of cancer.

High Cholesterol

Mangoes have high levels of soluble fiber, pectin and vitamin C, all of which help to lower serum cholesterol levels, especially LDL cholesterol (the bad cholesterol). Research suggests that compounds in mangoes could ease the effects of high cholesterol.

Low Sex Drive

Mangoes are rich in vitamins C and E. Vitamin E has been proven to regulate sex hormones and boost sex drive. In addition, research conducted at the University of Maryland Medical Center suggests that vitamin C can help with sexual problems such erectile dysfunction and a low libido.

Skin Problems

If you suffer from skin problems, you may want to think about adding mangoes to your diet. Applying mangoes directly to the skin will help to get rid of clogged pores, however eating mangoes regularly helps to reduce dry skin and flakiness, leaving the skin soft and shining from the inside out.

Olives

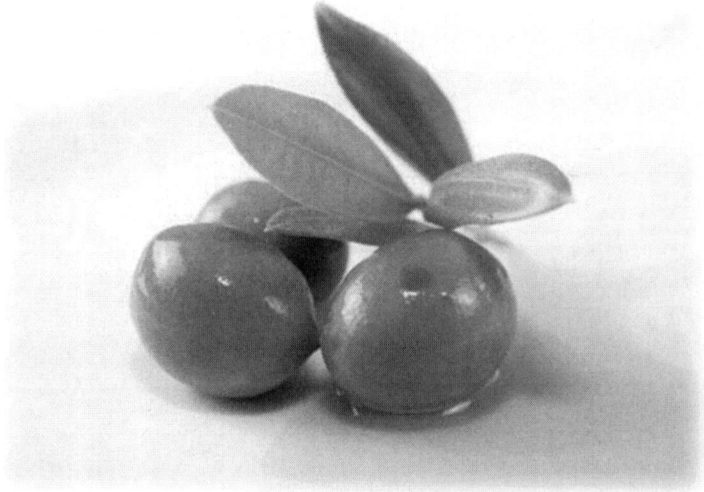

Although we generally think of olives as a zesty vegetable, they are technically classified as a fruit. Olives are nothing short of astounding. Few high-fat foods offer such a diverse range of valuable antioxidant and anti-inflammatory nutrients. Olives provide almost three-quarters of their fat as oleic acid, a healthy monounsaturated fatty acid, and offer us dozens of protective health benefits.

Bone Loss

Hydroxytyrosol is a phytonutrient in olive oil that has been found to have the potential to help us prevent bone loss. Several studies have found increased depositing of calcium in bone and decreased loss of total bone mass following consumption of this olive phytonutrient.

Cancer

Olives are a great source of vitamin E and monounsaturated fat, which have the ability to neutralize free radicals in the body. If our cells get overwhelmed by oxidative stress caused by free radicals and chronic excessive inflammation, our risk of cancer is increased. By providing us with rich supplies of antioxidant and anti-inflammatory nutrients, olives can help us avoid this dangerous combination of chronic oxidative stress and chronic inflammation.

Studies have shown that olive oil exerts a protective effect against certain malignant tumors in the breast, prostate, and digestive tract. Olive oil rich diets have been shown to reduce the number of cancerous lesions, result in less aggressive tumors and a better prognosis.

Heart Disease

Oleuropein is found exclusively in olives and has been shown to decrease oxidation of LDL cholesterol. In addition, the high monounsaturated fat content of olives has been associated with reduced risk of cardiovascular disease and decreased blood pressure. The oleic acid found in olives affects changes at cell membrane levels which result in decreased blood pressure.

Inflammation

The monounsaturated fats, vitamin E, and polyphenols in olive oil have anti-inflammatory abilities. Olive oil also contains a chemical called oleocanthal, which acts as a painkiller and inhibits inflammation by the same means that drugs like Ibuprofen do.

Orange

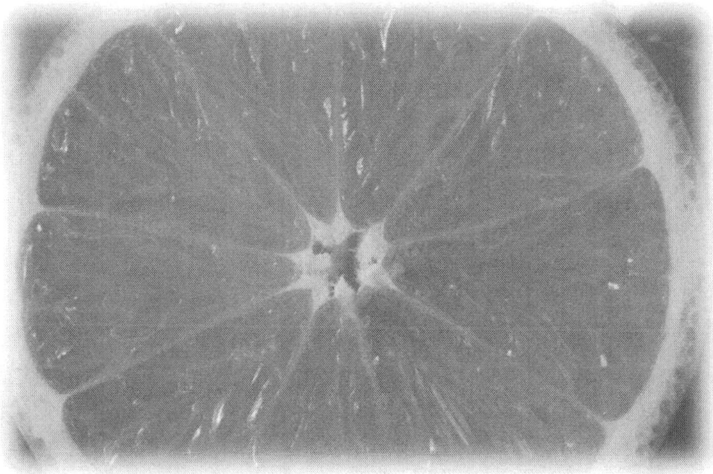

Oranges have many health benefits. They are packed with vitamins C and A, flavonoids, antioxidants, calcium, magnesium, potassium, dietary fiber.

Asthma Inflammation

Asthma is a chronic inflammatory lung disease that causes wheezing, difficulty breathing and chest tightness. Asthma symptoms can be triggered by allergens such as pollen or pet dander and by non-allergic triggers such as emotional stress, physical activity, cold air, smoke, or viruses. Consuming oranges and other citrus fruits may help reduce your symptoms. Citrus fruits are rich sources of vitamin A and C which help lessen lung inflammation associated with cigarette smoke and other pollutants.

Chest Congestion

Chest congestion can make breathing difficult and can cause coughing and shortness of breath. Oranges have an effect on the secretion of mucus by the glands lining your respiratory system. Oranges are also rich in vitamin C which is an essential nutrient that may help increase the effectiveness of your immune system. This can help reduce the severity and duration of conditions that cause chest congestion. Foods that are rich in vitamin C also tend to be a natural source of water, which can help reduce the thickness of mucus.

Papaya

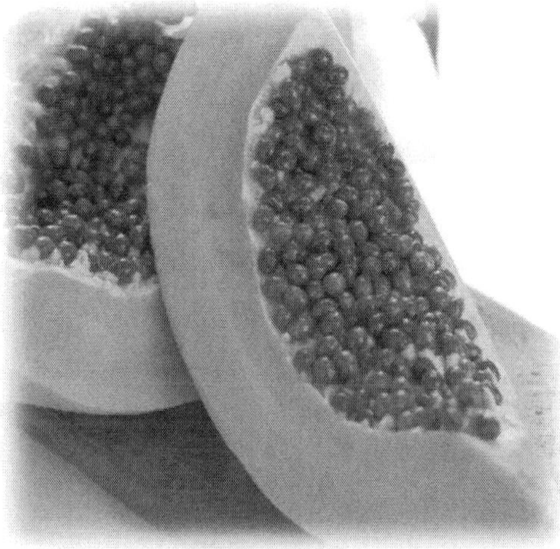

Papayas are rich in antioxidants, phytonutrients, vitamins, minerals, and special digestive enzymes that have a remarkable effect on proper digestion and overall health.

Cancer

Cancer is one of the world's leading killers. Papaya can be very beneficial for reducing your risk of developing certain types of cancers. Studies suggest that the proteolytic enzymes in papaya can digest the fibrin protein layer of cancer cells that usually surrounds and protects them, leaving the cancerous cells more susceptible to the body's immune response. Papayas also contain isothiocyanates which may help prevent cancer by eliminating potential carcinogens from our bodies and enhancing the action of tumor suppressing proteins and lycopene, which research has shown to have anticancer properties.

Gastrointestinal Problems

Undigested proteins can lead to many health issues, such as gastrointestinal problems and an overgrowth of flatulence causing bacteria in the colon. The primary therapeutic enzyme in papayas, papain, is a cysteine protease enzyme that is well known for its various digestive health benefits. Papayas improve digestion by breaking down proteins into their individual amino acids and dissolving fats. Its anti-inflammatory effects also help to soothe upset stomach.

Wrinkles

Papayas are a great source of antioxidant vitamins C and E and carotenoids, nutrients which can help protect your skin against free radicals known to cause damage that leads to wrinkles and signs of aging. Papayas also contain enzymes that help to soften the texture of the skin by dissolving some fats from under the skin.

Pineapple

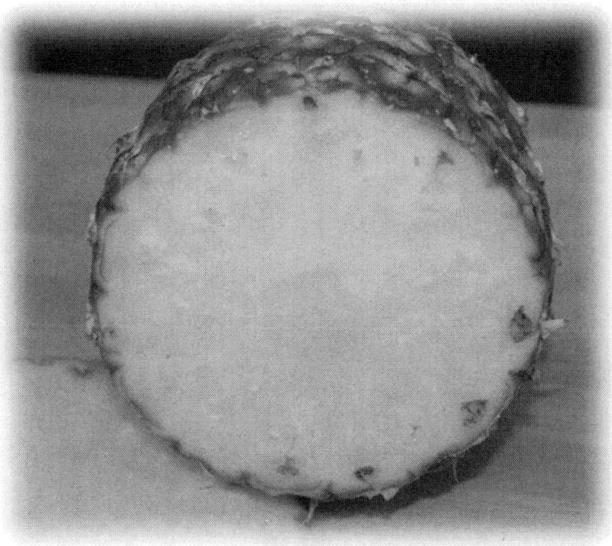

Pineapples are sweet, juicy, and delicious, but more importantly, they are very healthy and nutritious. Pineapples are loaded with vitamins and minerals including vitamin A, vitamin C, calcium, phosphorus, and potassium. Papayas are also rich in fiber.

Asthma Inflammation

The bromelain in pineapple has been shown to reduce asthma inflammation. Studies have found that bromelain can significantly reduce markers of lung inflammation and reduce the total white blood cells which normally increase with the onset of asthma.

Warning: While pineapples can be beneficial for asthma inflammation, it is important to remember that not all treatments work the same for everyone. Asthma attacks can be life threatening; for your own safety, please speak to your doctor before initiating any alternative asthma therapy and/or discontinuing your use of prescription medications.

Gastrointestinal Problems

Suffering from gastrointestinal or digestive problems is not fun. Pineapples are one of the best foods to help promote healthy digestion and ease gastrointestinal problems. Pineapples can help us avoid digestive problems like gas, bloating, upset stomach, diarrhea, burping and constipation. The bromelain in pineapple improves digestion by breaking down hard to digest proteins into their individual amino acids. Pineapples are also rich in fiber which offers additional digestive benefits.

Pomegranate

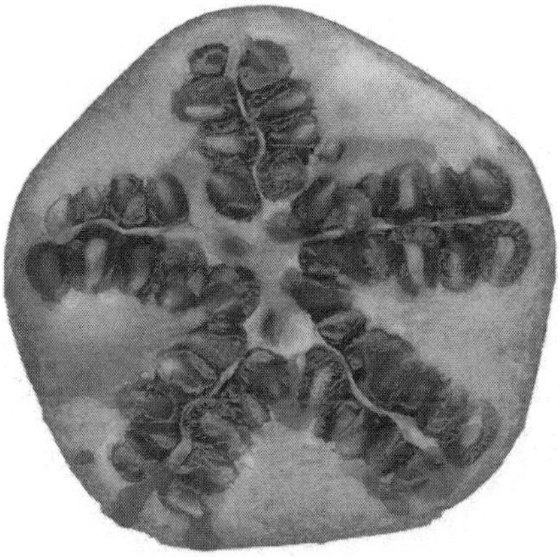

This nutrient dense, antioxidant rich fruit has been revered as a symbol of health throughout history. Punicalagins, compounds only founds in pomegranates, are mostly responsible for the pomegranate's health benefits. One glass of pomegranate juice has more antioxidants than red wine, green tea, and blueberries.

Heart Disease

The potent antioxidant compounds in pomegranates have been shown to reduce platelet aggregation, reduce atherosclerosis, and lower blood pressure. A recent medical study published in the journal of *Clinical Nutrition* found that patients with severe carotid artery blockages who drank a glass a pomegranate juice every day for a year saw a 12% reduction in blood pressure and a 30% reduction in atherosclerotic plaque. Pomegranates contain high levels of flavonoids and polyphenols, potent antioxidants that protect against heart disease.

Low Sex Drive

Want to boost your sex drive? Pomegranates have been shown to increase sex drive. Studies indicate that drinking pomegranate juice daily for 2 weeks can elevate levels of sexual interest in both men and women by increasing their levels of testosterone. Pomegranates also help the body produce nitric oxide which helps to open up blood vessels and increase to blood flow which in turns increases libido.

Tomato

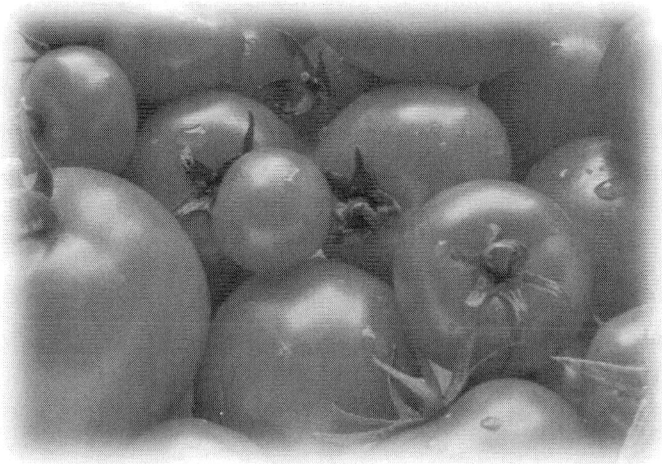

Botanically classified as a fruit, tomatoes are sweet, juicy, and delicious. Tomatoes are not only a tasty addition to salads, but they are packed with nutritional benefits as well. Tomatoes are a good source of vitamins A, C and K, folate, and potassium, and also provide thiamin, niacin, vitamin B6, magnesium, phosphorus, and copper, all of which are necessary for good health. They are naturally low in calories, fat, cholesterol, and sodium.

Cancer

Tomatoes are a natural cancer fighter. Lycopene is rare in foods, and tomatoes are one of only a few foods that are naturally rich in this powerful antioxidant. Clinical studies have shown that lycopene can reduce the risk of cancers such as prostate, cervical, mouth, throat, stomach, colon, rectal, prostate, and ovarian cancer. In addition, the vitamin A and C in tomatoes fight the free radicals which can cause cell damage. Ironically, processed tomatoes (sauce, paste, etc.) are more effective than raw tomatoes at reducing cancer risk. The processing breaks down the cell walls which trap the lycopene making it more bioavailable. Tomatoes have been shown to be particularly effective against prostate cancers.

Eye Conditions

The vitamin A that tomatoes provide can improve vision and help prevent eye conditions such as night blindness and macular degeneration. A deficiency in vitamin A contributes to the development of night blindness. A one cup serving of fresh tomatoes provides 30% of the daily value of vitamin A.

Osteoporosis

Tomatoes build strong bones and can ward off osteoporosis. Lycopene slows down the breakdown of bone cells and the vitamin K and calcium in tomatoes help strengthen and repair bones. A serving of tomatoes provides 18% the daily value for vitamin K.

VEGETABLES

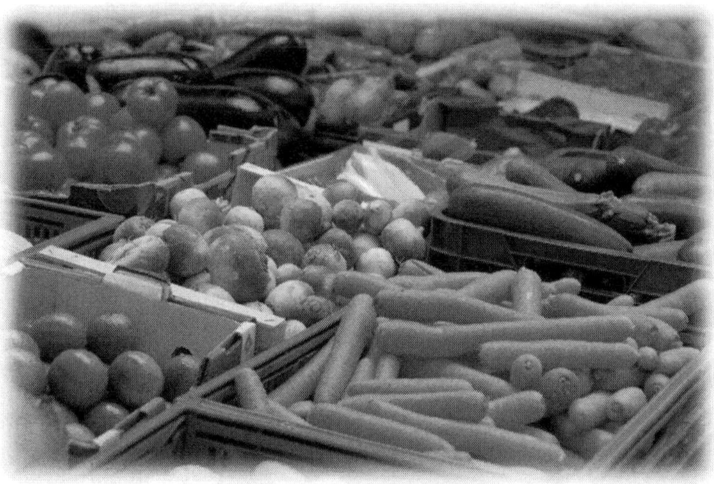

Preserve and treat food as you would your body,
remembering that in time food will be your body.
—B.W. Richardson

While the health-related benefits of a diet rich in vegetables is known to most, scientific research has increasingly pointed to their influence on a variety of diseases. Like fruits, vegetables are loaded with vitamins and mineral including phytonutrients and antioxidants such as vitamin A, C, E, and selenium. Options like broccoli, tomatoes, spinach provide additional benefits. People who eat more vegetables as part of an overall healthy diet are likely to have a reduced risk of many chronic diseases.

Asparagus

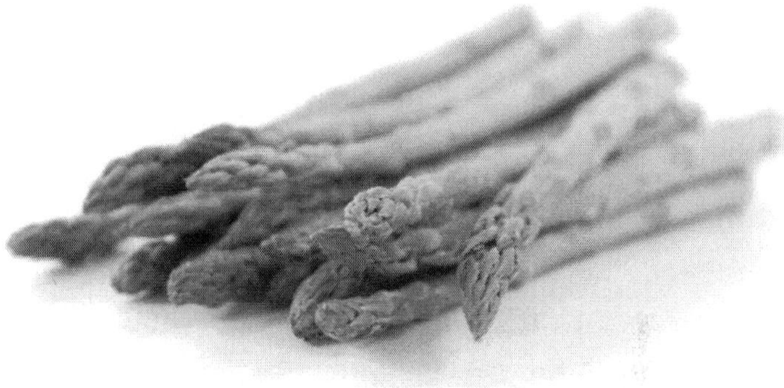

Asparagus is a very good source of fiber, folate, vitamins A, C, E and K, and chromium. They are also a good source of anti-oxidants such as lutein, zeaxanthin, carotenes, and cryptoxanthins.

Cancer

Asparagus is packed with antioxidants which help neutralize cell-damaging free radicals. Asparagus is the best food source of glutathione, a detoxifying compound that helps break down carcinogens and other harmful compounds. In addition, Asparin A, a compound in asparagus, has been found to halt the growth of liver cancer cells and can even cause death in those cells. Chronic inflammation and oxidative stress are risk factors for a variety of cancer types. The steroidal glycosides compounds in asparagus have strong anti-inflammatory and antioxidant properties.

Weight Loss

Asparagus has an exceptionally high nutrient/calorie ratio and may be the perfect weight-loss food. Asparagus is a rich source of the soluble fiber inulin, which has been shown to suppress appetite. Asparagus is also a very low calorie food. In fact, asparagus is a negative calorie food, which means that more calories are burned digesting it than it provides. Asparagus also helps to maintain your blood sugar levels stable which can help you avoid crashes and binges that lead to overeating.

Artichoke

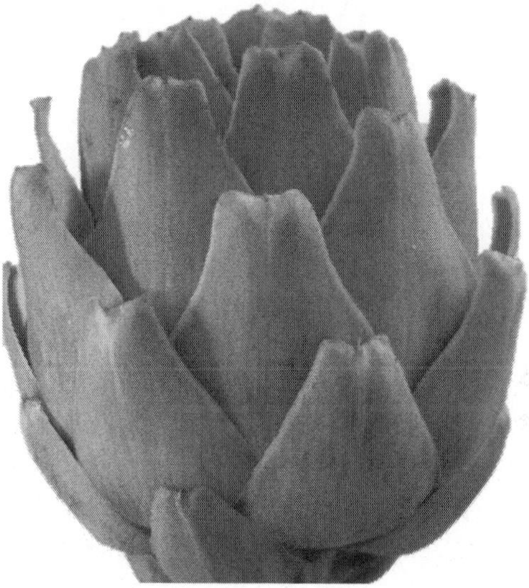

Artichokes have one of the highest levels of antioxidants. Some of the powerful antioxidants in artichokes are quercetin, rutin, anthocyanins, cynarin, luteolin, and silymarin. Artichokes are low in calories and are a great source of dietary fiber.

High Blood Glucose Levels

An artichoke has a glycemic index ranking of 15, which places it among the very lowest foods or beverages on the glycemic index. Scientific evidence shows that the artichoke can help balance blood glucose levels. Glycogen is stored in the body and turned into sugar whenever blood sugar supplies are low. The overproduction of glucose by the liver can lead to diabetes and other health problems. The cynarin present in artichokes can keep the liver from producing too much glucose.

Liver Ailments

Few veggies are as potent as the artichoke in helping an ailing liver. Studies have found they may even regenerate liver tissue. Experts believe that artichokes help stimulate production of bile in the liver as well as promote the movement of bile through the system. These two functions are vital to the liver's well-being. One of the jobs of bile is to remove toxins through the bowel. If bile is not transported adequately, the liver has an increased risk of being damaged. It has been suggested that 30 minutes after eating globe artichoke, bile flow is increased by over 100%. Artichokes have long been used in folk and alternative medicine as a treatment for liver ailments and the scientific studies are now proving them to be correct.

Beets

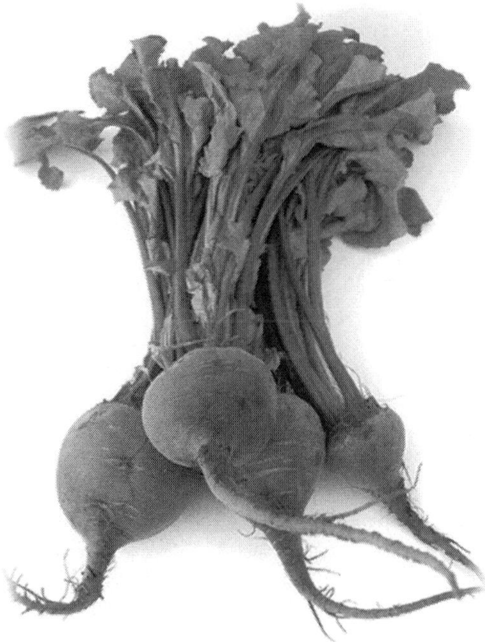

Beets are one of those often overlooked foods, but adding beets to your diet can greatly increase your well-being and immunity. The roots and leaves of the beet have long been used to treat a wide variety of ailments.

Anemia

Anemia is a condition in which too few red blood cells are in circulation. Iron deficiency is the most frequent cause of anemia. Beets are good source of iron which regenerates and reactivates the red blood cells and supplies fresh oxygen to the body. The copper content in beets helps make the iron more available to the body.

Depression

Depression, mental fatigue, and insomnia have been linked with lower levels of folate. One cup of beets supplies you with 30% of your daily needs. Beets contain trimethylglycine, the same substance that is used in certain treatments of depression. It also contains tryptophan, which relaxes the mind and creates a sense of well-being.

Erectile Dysfunction

Some foods increase circulation because of their high concentration of nitrates. Beets contain a high amount of nitrate which causes dilation of the blood cells allowing more blood to get around the veins. Nitrates have been shown to have beneficial effects for erectile dysfunction. Prescription ED medications are based on the relaxing effects of nitrates on the blood vessels that supply the penis.

Heart Disease

The beet is one of the best sources of both folate and betaine. These two nutrients help to lower your blood levels of homocysteine, an inflammatory compound that can damage your arteries and increase your risk of heart disease. It also helps to keep the blood vessels and the arterial system in a very sound condition. The juice of this wonderful root is a powerful solvent for inorganic calcium deposits that cause the arteries to harden and therefore it is very useful in fighting arteriosclerosis.

Poor Circulation

Beet juice is best known as a blood purifier and blood builder that help in the creation of red blood cells. Beet juice can help in the construction of red blood cells which help to carry oxygen around the body. Beets contain nitrate which causes dilation of the blood cells allowing more blood to get around the veins thereby reducing high blood pressure. This then improves circulation.

Broccoli

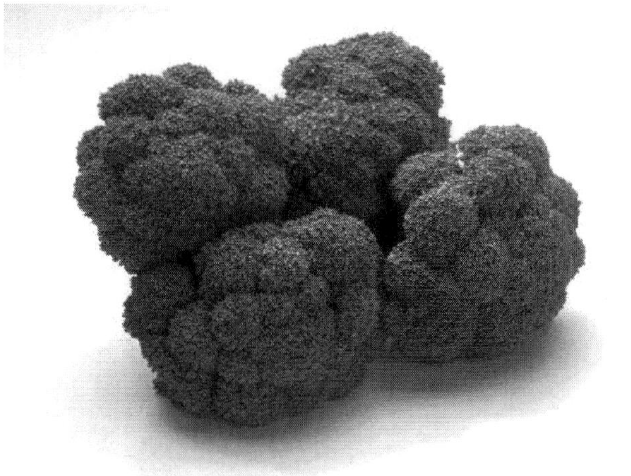

Some people love broccoli and others hate it, but there's no denying that broccoli is a nutritional powerhouse. Broccoli is an excellent source of vitamins C, K, and A, as well as folate and dietary fiber, and a very good source of manganese, potassium, magnesium, and phosphorus, and vitamins B2 and B6. In addition to providing these valuable nutrients, broccoli offers an abundance of powerful phytochemicals that may help protect the body against many ailments including cancers.

Blood Pressure

Research indicates that glucoraphanin, a compound found in broccoli, may reduce the risk of high blood pressure. Broccoli also contains potassium, magnesium, and calcium which also help regulate blood pressure.

Cancer

Diets high in broccoli have been linked with a lower risk of certain types of cancer. Broccoli contains certain chemicals that work through numerous mechanisms to inhibit tumor cell adhesion, spread, and invasion. These substances act as antioxidants, boost detoxifying enzymes in the body, and may even produce beneficial changes in gene expression. Studies suggest that a broccoli compound known as sulforaphane induces cancer cells to commit a sort of cellular suicide.

Liver Ailments

The liver is one of the most important organs of the body. It is responsible for regulating blood sugar, absorbing nutrients, and eliminating harmful substances from the body. Broccoli is a very powerful detoxifier of the liver. Broccoli increases the amount of glucosinolate which helps the liver to produce the enzymes it needs for its detoxification processes. Broccoli also contains chemicals that neutralize certain toxins.

Carrots

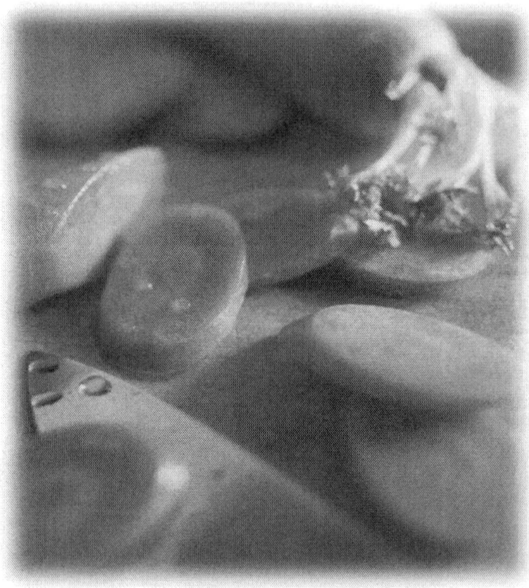

Everyone knows that carrots are great for eyesight, but your vision isn't the only thing carrots are good for. Carrots are an excellent source of various essential nutrients and have many other health benefits.

Asthma Inflammation

Carrots are a top source for beta-carotene, hence the name. Beta-carotene may reduce lung inflammation caused by toxins and may also decrease asthma symptoms caused by exercise.

Cancer

Carrots contain numerous powerful cancer-fighting antioxidants and vitamins. Various studies have shown that carrots may help lower the risk of breast, colon, and lung cancer. Studies have shown that women who regularly consume carrots have a lower chance of suffering from cancer than those who rarely eat carrots. Carrots contain Retinoic acid which is efficient in fighting against breast cancer in the early stages. Carrots are rich in carotenoids, hence the name. Carotenoids are very beneficial as they fight off oxygen free radicals that are principally responsible for cancer growth and development. Falcarinol, a compound in carrots that protects carrots from fungal diseases, is also responsible for many of the carrot's anticancer benefits.

Heart Disease

Diets high in carrots are associated with a lower risk of heart disease. Carrots are high in fiber and beta-carotene; nutrients which help keep blood pressure down and reduce cholesterol levels, thus reducing the risk of heart disease. Studies indicate that consuming about 2 baby carrots daily can lower the risk of coronary heart disease by approximately 32%.

Vision Problems

Carrots are rich in beta-carotene and lutein which are vital for eye health. Beta-carotene is an important precursor for vitamin A. Severe deficiencies in vitamin A can cause blindness. Beta-carotene helps to protect against macular degeneration and against the development of senile cataracts. Studies have found that people who eat plenty of carrots have a much lower risk of macular degeneration than those who eat very little.

Spinach

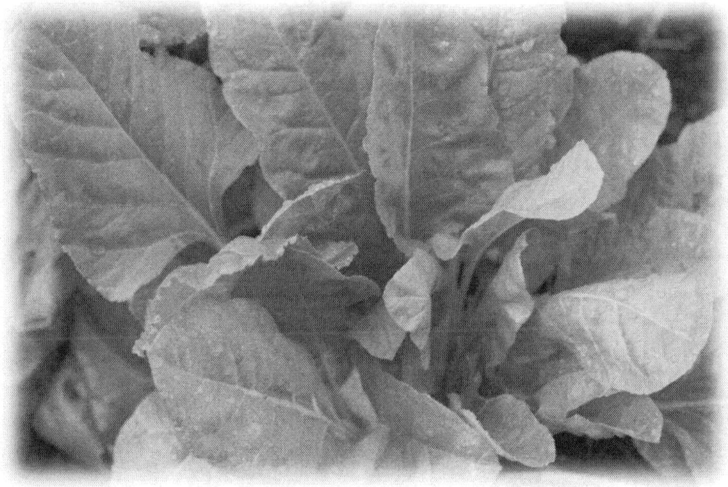

Spinach is a nutritional powerhouse. It is one of the most nutrient dense foods in existence. Spinach is packed with vitamin C, vitamin E, beta-carotene, manganese, zinc, and selenium which all serve as powerful antioxidants that protect against many diseases and health conditions.

Dull Hair

Spinach is excellent for overall hair health and shine. Spinach is loaded with vitamins A and C, which help your body to create sebum, the oil secreted by follicles to give your hair gloss and shine.

High Blood Pressure

Spinach is low in calories, high in fiber, and packed with heart-healthy nutrients like potassium, folate, and magnesium. Magnesium is essential in maintaining healthy levels of blood pressure. In fact, just a salad-size portion of spinach will work to lower high blood pressure within hours.

Osteoporosis

One cup of cooked spinach provides over 1000% of the daily recommended vitamin K which helps prevent excess activation of osteoclasts, the cells that break down bones. Vitamin K also promotes the synthesis of osteocalcin, an essential protein for maintaining the strength and density of our bones.

Restless Leg Syndrome

Those who experience Restless Leg Syndrome (RLS) have difficulty getting a good night's sleep because they are seized by uncontrollable urge to move their legs while in bed. Because RLS often results in sleep deprivation, it can lead to anxiety and depression. RLS has been associated with low levels of iron, magnesium and folate. Foods high in these nutrients have been shown to be helpful in easing the symptoms of RLS. Spinach is rich in folate, iron, and magnesium.

HERBS AND SPICES

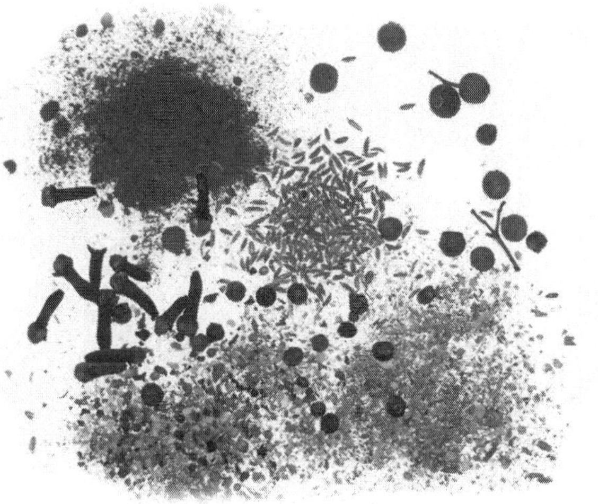

He who distinguishes the true savor of his food can never be a glutton; he who does not cannot be otherwise.
—Henry David Thoreau

Herbs and spices can benefit your health as much as they do your taste buds. Herbs and spices are teeming with healthy antioxidants and phytonutrients. They have more disease fighting antioxidants than many fruits and vegetables.

Cinnamon

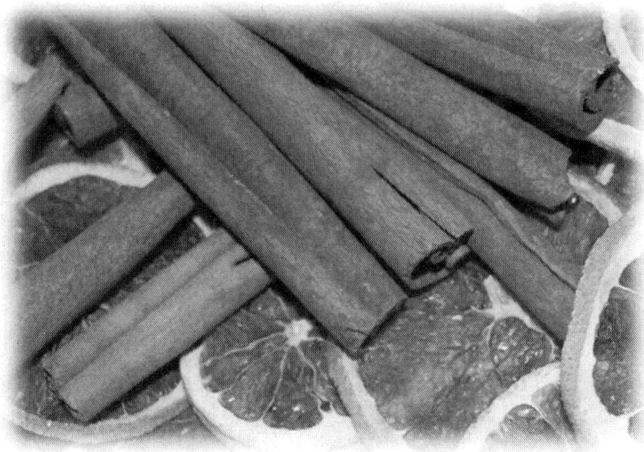

Who doesn't love to sprinkle a little cinnamon on oatmeal or morning latte? Cinnamon is not only tasty, but it is also quite beneficial to our health.

High Blood Sugar

Cinnamon has been shown to be of great value in maintaining healthy blood sugar levels. Cinnamon mimics the effects of insulin and has a regulatory effect on blood sugar, making it especially beneficial for people with Type 2 diabetes. The American Diabetes Association has found that taking 3 to 6 grams of cinnamon per day can lower glucose levels in people with Type 2 diabetes. A recent study published in the *American Journal of*

Clinical Nutrition found that consuming about teaspoon of cinnamon even helped tame blood sugar in people without diabetes.

High Cholesterol

Cinnamon contains polyphenols which create healthier arteries and reduce the risk of cardiovascular disease. Scientists have found evidence that cinnamon helps lower lipid levels. Just ½ teaspoon of cinnamon per day may help you lower triglycerides and LDL cholesterol levels.

Garlic

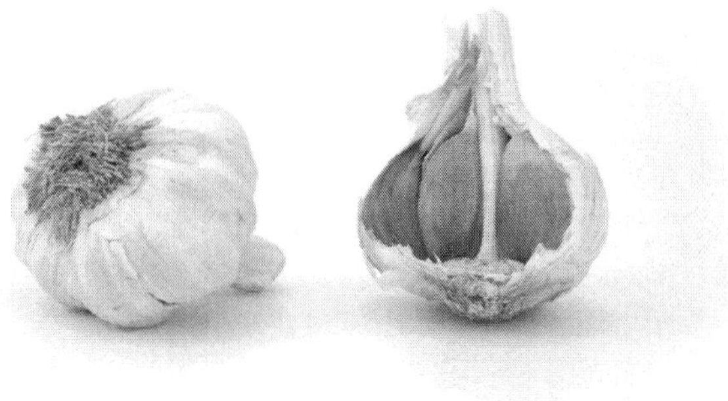

People have known for centuries that garlic has many healing properties and it has been used throughout recorded history for its medicinal (as well culinary) uses.

Cancer

Several studies have shown a link between increased garlic intake and reduced risk of certain cancers, including cancers of the stomach, colon, esophagus, pancreas, and breast. Another study showed that women who ate the most garlic had a 50% lower risk of cancer of the colon compared with women who ate the least.

Candidiasis

Candida is a fungus that causes candidiasis; or what is more commonly known as a yeast infection. We all have some amount of yeast on our skin and in our bodies, but when an overgrowth of yeast occurs, we can experience very unpleasant symptoms; this overgrowth of yeast is referred to as a yeast infection or candidiasis. Most yeast infections occur in the vagina, as a diaper rash in young children, as thrush in nursing infants, or as skin infections in people with a compromised immune system. Garlic can be an effective treatment for candidiasis. Crushed garlic contains allicin which has anti-bacterial and anti-fungal properties.

Erectile Dysfunction

In order to maintain an erection, the arteries need to have an efficient blood flow. Crushed garlic contains allicin, a compound that can decrease blood pressure and improve blood flow, which may lead to a harder erection.

Infections

Garlic contains allicin which is a powerful antibiotic and a potent agent that helps the body to inhibit the ability of germs to grow and reproduce. Garlic has been used effectively against a whole host of bacteria, fungus, and viruses. Some studies suggest that garlic is an even more powerful germ-killer than either penicillin or tetracycline.

Liver Ailments

A healthy liver maintains blood flow and circulation, breaking down nutrients from foods and distributing them to other body organs. Garlic contains allicin which is a sulphur-based compound needed by the liver for effective detoxification. The antioxidants in garlic help keep toxic substances filtered by your liver from reaching other organs. Garlic has been shown to help the liver rid the body of mercury, food additives, and the hormone estrogen.

> *Warning: Although garlic is generally considered safe so it would be difficult to overdose on it. However, garlic has properties that can be dangerous if you suffer from a clotting disorder.*

Hot Peppers

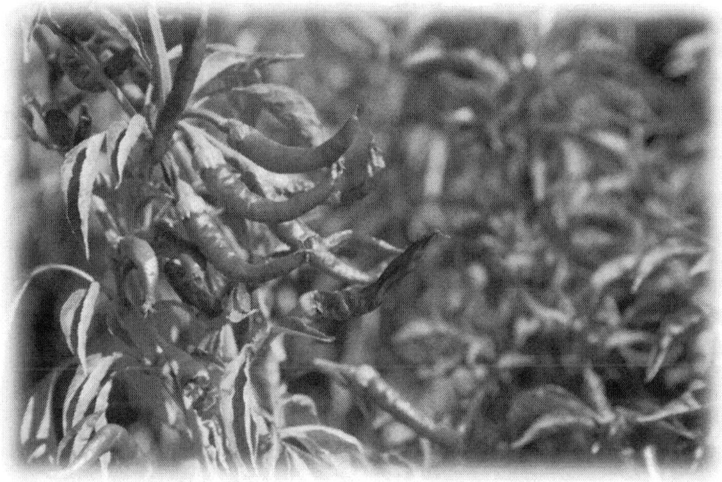

Some people just can't get enough of the painful pleasure of hot spicy foods. Fortunately, capsaicin, the compound that gives hot peppers like habaneros and jalapeños their kick, has many proven health benefits. Capsaicin is a flavorless, odorless, colorless compound found in varying amounts in peppers. The hotter the pepper, the more capsaicin it contains and the higher amount of health improving antioxidants.

Heart Disease

Hot peppers are a heart healthy food. The compounds in hot peppers, including capsaicin, have been found to lower blood pressure, decrease cholesterol levels, and reduce the risk for dangerous blood clots.

Pain

Capsaicin, the active ingredient in hot peppers, has been shown to reduce pain. It acts by binding to receptors in the cell wall of nerve endings and triggering an influx of calcium ions into the neurons. It also interferes with substance P, a chemical involved in transmitting pain impulses to the brain.

Parsley

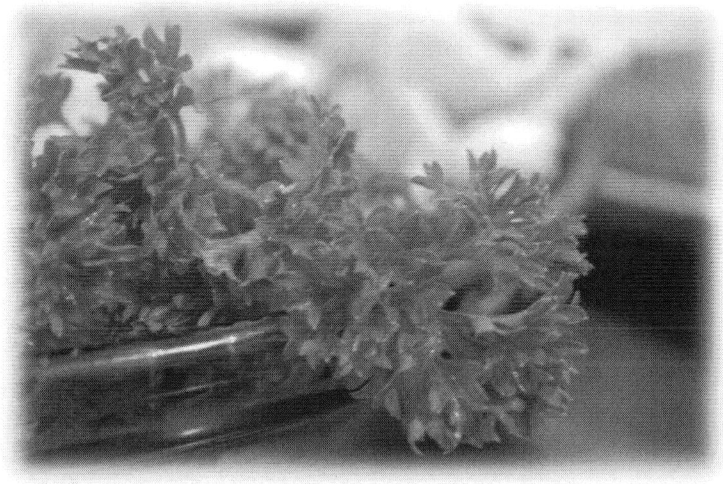

Though traditionally overlooked as just a garnish, parsley has various health benefits. Parsley is rich in antioxidants including luteolin, a flavonoid that searches out and eradicates free radicals in the body that cause oxidative stress in cells. Luteolin also promotes carbohydrate metabolism. Parsley is rich in many essential vitamins, including vitamins A and C, B 12, and K.

Halitosis

Bad breath can be an embarrassing nuisance especially in social situations. Parsley contains chemicals that help to freshen bad breath. Parsley is rich in chlorophyll which has antioxidant and anti-inflammatory properties and helps to neutralize toxins and pollutants and act as a natural deodorizer. Chewing a small handful of parsley allows you to gain the breath-freshening benefits of chlorophyll. This may be the reason why parsley makes an appearance as a garnish on so many restaurant dishes.

Thyme

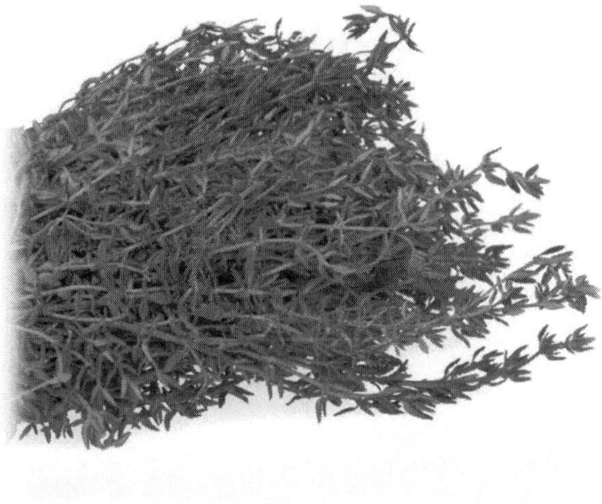

Thyme is credited with many virtues. This fragrant herb has been used since ancient times for medicinal and culinary uses. Thyme contains thymol and the antioxidant flavonoids apigenin, naringenin, luteolin, and thymonin.

Coughs

The next time you have a cold or cough, try a cup of thyme tea. Thyme has been shown to have bronchodilating and antispasmodic effects, so it helps to relax the bronchial tubes and alleviates coughing fits. Thyme oil is used in many cough syrups because it acts as an expectorant loosening mucous and has antibacterial and antiseptic properties.

Gas and Indigestion

Thyme is often recommended to promote good digestion and relieve gas and bloating. The volatile oils in thyme help reduce gas while its phenols work as an antispasmodic, helping to relieve intestinal cramping.

NUTS AND SEEDS

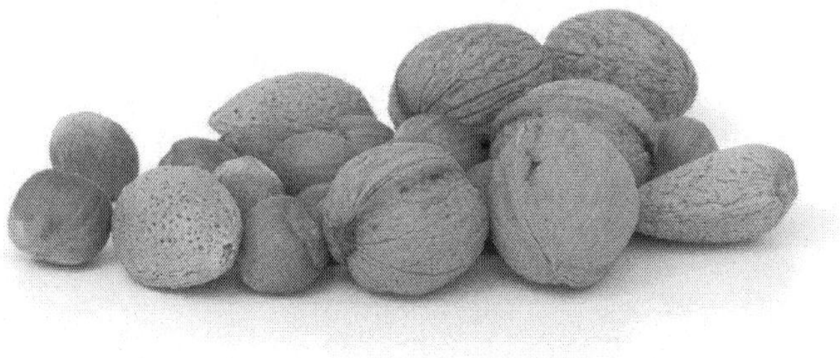

If we're not willing to settle for junk living, we certainly shouldn't settle for junk food.
—Sally Edwards

If nuts are not part of your regular snack choices, then you are missing out on some major disease-fighting nutrients that protect your heart, boost mental power, and more. Just a handful of nuts a day will help you to stay healthy and fit. Nuts are rich in antioxidants, protein, vitamins, minerals, and omega-3 fatty acids. Nuts are a crunchy and delicious alternative to traditional junk food snacks.

Almond

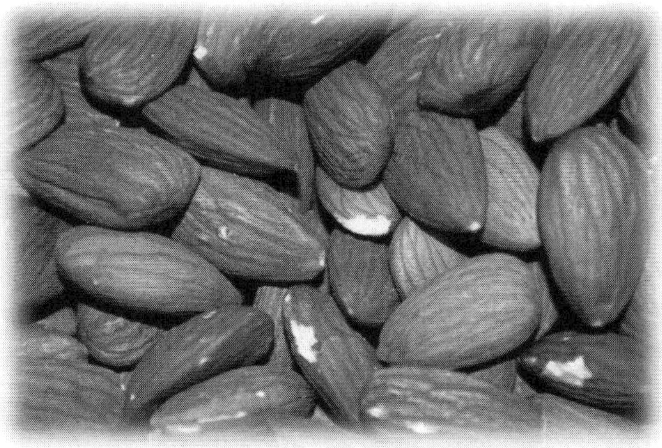

Almonds are a wonderfully delicious snack. Almonds have long been revered as the promoter of wellness and health. Almonds are high in fiber, vitamin E, powerful antioxidants.

High Cholesterol

Almonds are rich in dietary fiber, vitamins, and minerals, and are packed with numerous health promoting phytochemicals. Almonds contain unsaturated fatty acids like oleic and palmitoleic acids which have been shown to lower blood LDL (bad cholesterol) and increase HDL (good cholesterol) levels and thus helping to prevent coronary artery disease and strokes.

Brazil Nut

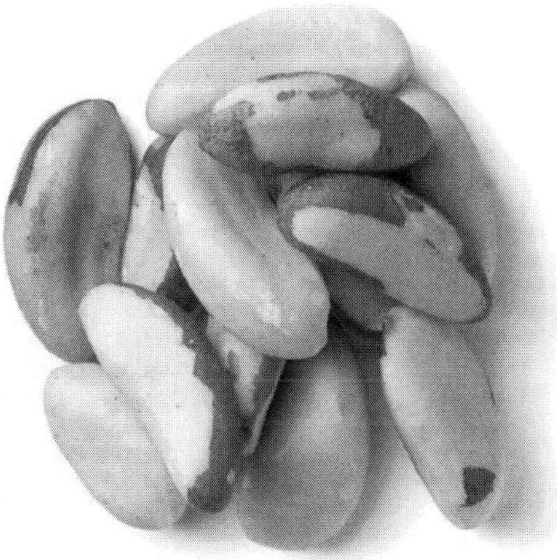

Brazil nuts are extremely tasty treats and are loaded with health benefits. They contain exceptionally high levels of selenium. Just 1 ounce of these nuts provides about 800% of the recommended daily intake of selenium making them the highest natural source of this mineral. High levels of selenium are associated with many health benefits.

Heart Disease

Selenium is a very powerful and essential nutrient. It encourages the production of glutathione, an important antioxidant that helps protect our body from free radical damage. Selenium helps prevent blood clotting and protect us from heart disease and strokes. Studies have shown that higher concentrations of selenium in the blood are associated with reduced risk of coronary heart disease.

Cacao (Raw Chocolate!)

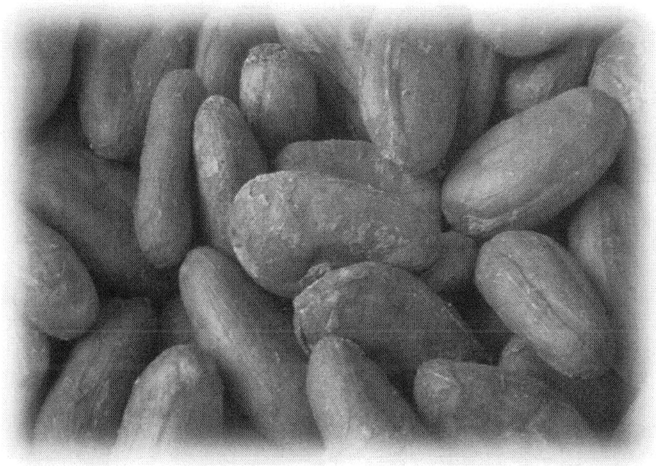

The cacao nut (raw chocolate) is packed with a myriad of beneficial properties including minerals, vitamins, antioxidants, Theobromine, Phenylethylamine.

Depression and Mood

Cacao is a mood enhancer. Phenylethylamine, in combination with theobromine, can elevate mood and create a sense well-being. Eating cacao can raise your natural levels of serotonin and create a balancing effect.

PMS

Cacao is a very rich source of magnesium. Magnesium balances brain chemistry and has a strong influence on feelings of well-being and happiness. If you suffer from PMS, your levels of serotonin are likely low. This is probably the main reason why many women crave chocolate during the monthly cycle; eating chocolate or cacao seeds can raise your levels of serotonin.

Flaxseeds

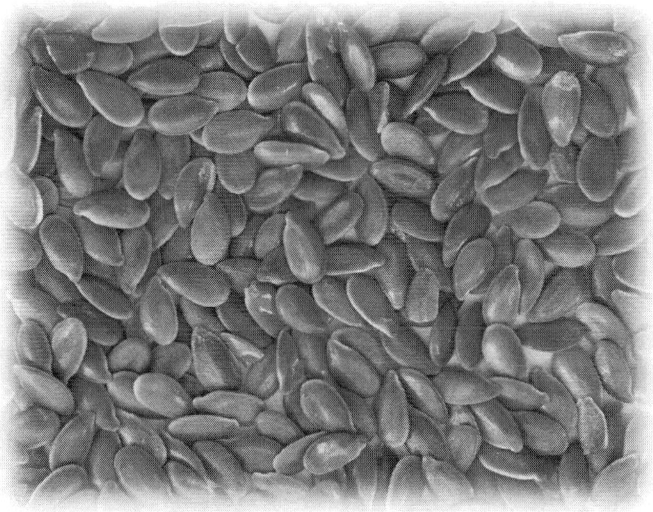

Flax seeds are a nutrient dense power food. Flax seeds are rich in B vitamins, magnesium, manganese, and omega-3 fatty acids.

Cognitive Problems

Flax seeds are rich in brain-healthy fats including omega-3 fatty acids which are directly used by the brain to build and protect neurons. Flax seeds also contain GLA, an omega-6 fatty acid which are used to build healthy neurons and also to regulate the environment of the brain. To boost your brain power to the max, have a tablespoon or two of flax seeds every day.

Constipation

Everyone experiences a bout of constipation now and then. Constipation is often simply the result of consuming too little fiber, and adding more fiber to your diet is the simple remedy. Flax seed are high in fiber. You'd be hard-pressed to find a food higher in fiber than flax.

GRAINS AND LEGUMES

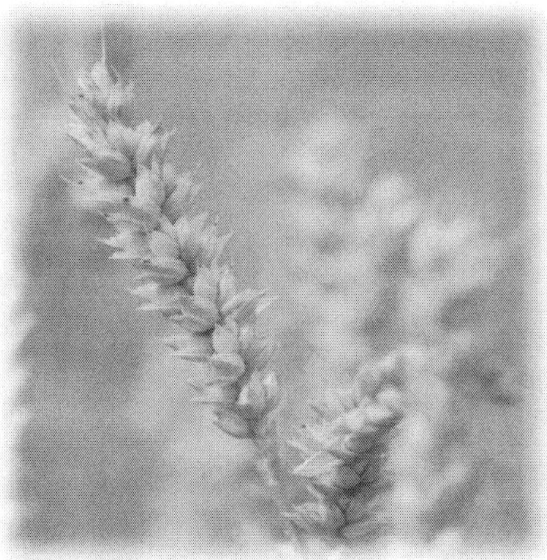

Courage, cheerfulness, and a desire to work depend mostly on good nutrition.
—Jacob Moleschott

Whole grains can be important part of a healthy diet. Consuming at least three servings of whole grains per day can reduce the risk of chronic health conditions like cardiovascular disease and Type II diabetes. Eating whole grains instead of refined grains can reduce the potential for excess abdominal fat buildup, which can raise blood pressure and cholesterol levels, and even cause insulin resistance.

Oats

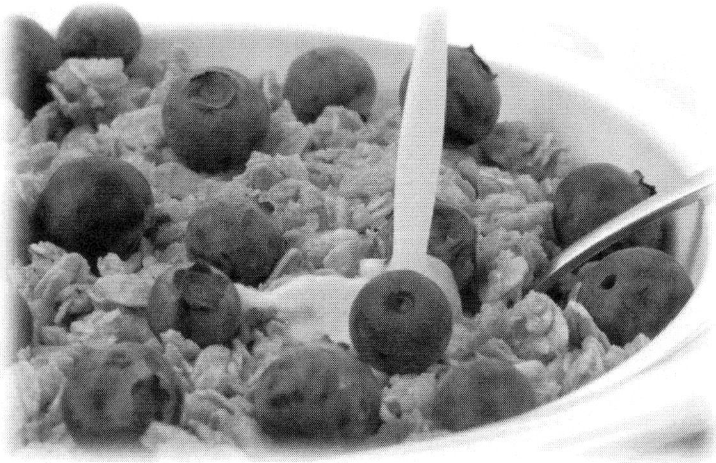

Nothing starts the day off better than a big bowl of warm oatmeal. The oat is generally cited as the most nourishing of all the cereals. Oats have a higher concentration of well-balanced protein than other cereals and contain phytochemicals which have been associated with protection from many forms of chronic disease. Oats also contain a good balance of essential fatty acids, which have been linked with longevity and general good health.

Heart Disease

The accumulation of cholesterol is implicated in many types of cardiovascular disease. Oatmeal and oat bran are significant sources of soluble and insoluble fiber. One component of the soluble fiber found in oats is beta-glucans, which has proven effective in lowering blood cholesterol. Oats are also one of the best sources of compounds called tocotrienols which inhibit cholesterol synthesis and have been found to lower blood cholesterol. Research also indicates that the antioxidants found in oats reduce cholesterol by reducing the ability of blood cells to stick to the inside of artery walls. A daily bowl of oatmeal can lower cholesterol by up to 23 percent and reduce the risk of heart disease by almost half.

Peanuts

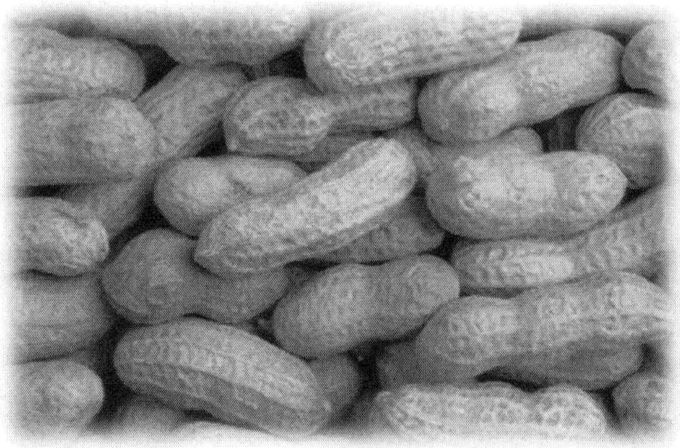

Although most think of peanuts as a nut, peanuts are really a legume (more like beans). Peanuts contain healthy fats, vitamins, minerals and other compounds that can help manage your risk of developing chronic diseases.

Anxiety

Gamma aminobutyric acid (GABA) is an atypical amino acid that acts as a neurotransmitter in your central nervous system. It has a calming effect and helps to reduce anxiety and nervousness. If you're not producing enough GABA, you are likely to feel anxious and nervous. Peanuts are one of the best sources of glutamine, the amino acid needed to make GABA.

PART III:
Health Conditions

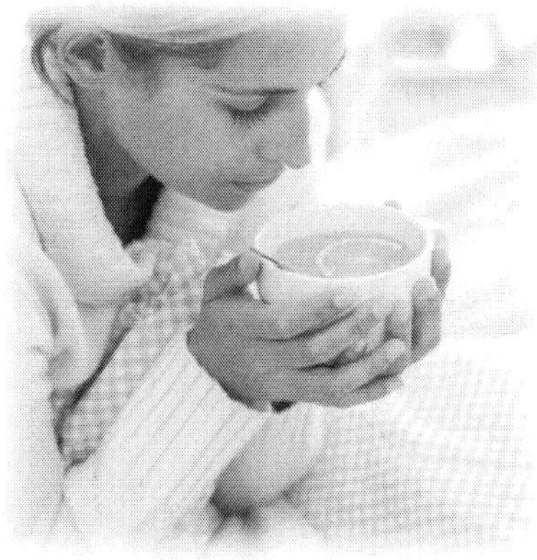

For every ailment under the sun, there is a remedy,
or there is none; if there be one, try to find it; if
there be none, never mind it.
—Mother Goose

This section is organized by health condition and is intended to serve as a cross reference to the information provided earlier in the book. Under each condition you will find the medicinal foods recommended or suggested for that particular condition. If you're tired of taking medications that only mask your symptoms, or worse, create new ones, it's time to start using the foods to heal your ailments.

Alzheimer's Disease

Alzheimer's is the most common form of dementia. It's a progressive disease that causes problems with memory, thinking and behavior. Unfortunately there is no cure for Alzheimer's. Although the clear causes of Alzheimer's disease are not yet well understood. Research indicates that the disease is associated with plaques and tangles in the brain. There are no available treatments that stop or reverse the progression of the disease and current treatments only help with the symptoms of the disease. Proper nutrition may decrease the risk, or slow the progression of Alzheimer's.

Apple

Eating apples can improve your memory and help you sustain overall brain health. Apples contain a larger percentage of phosphorus than any other fruit or vegetable. For this reason, it is an invaluable food for brain health. Sufferers of cognitive or memory problems should eat at least two apples every day. The effects of the antioxidants and flavonoids present in apples have been shown to reduce brain-cell inflammation and oxidation that occurs naturally due to the presence of free radicals. Eating apples increases acetylcholine, which is a critical neurotransmitter for memory and brain health. Eating apples has been shown to diminish accumulations of toxins in the brain, particularly beta-amyloid, which is thought to be one of the main factors causing Alzheimer's disease.

Blueberries

When it comes to brain health, there really is nothing quite like blueberries, some have even called them "brain berries." Blueberries are high in anthocyanins which help prevent the breakdown of brain cells. Studies have found that people who eat at least one cup of blueberries per week experience less mental decline compared to those who rarely eat them. In addition to anthocyanin, blueberries contain selenium, vitamins A, B-complex, C, and E, zinc, sodium, potassium, copper, magnesium, phosphorus, and manganese. These power-packed berries can help prevent degeneration and death of neurons and brain-cells and restore health of the central nervous system. Blueberries help protect the brain from oxidative stress and may reduce the effects of age-related memory impairments like dementia and Alzheimer's.

Acid Reflux

Acid reflux occurs when digestive fluid backs up past the lower esophageal sphincter into your esophagus. When this happens, you feel a burning pain in your chest or abdomen.

Mangoes

The tartaric acid, malic acid, and a trace of citric acid found in mangoes help to neutralize acid. The juice of the mango also coats the lining of the esophagus, relieving any pain caused by the acid moving upwards.

Acne

Acne occurs when skin cells, sebum and hair clump together plugging hair follicles which then become infected with bacteria, resulting in a swelling. While your instinct might be to run to the drugstore to purchase acne treatments, you can find an excellent treatment for your acne right in your refrigerator.

Lemon

Lemons have healing properties that work well to heal acne blemishes. Lemon juice can be applied directly to the skin or drunk as a beverage. Applied externally, lemons decrease inflammation, redness and irritation from acne and restore skin to health. Lemons are rich in vitamin C which has anti-inflammatory properties and alpha-hydroxy acid which works as a skin exfoliator. Lemons have disinfectant properties; the acid in lemon juice breaks down the main acne-causing bacteria, p. acnes. Internally, lemons works by stopping signals to the immune system to cause inflammation.

Anemia

Anemia is a condition in which too few red blood cells are in circulation. Iron deficiency is the most frequent cause of anemia.

Bananas

Bananas are high in iron which is essential for the production of hemoglobin, myoglobin, and enzymes essential in the production of red blood cells. They are therefore an excellent food for anemic persons.

Beets

Beets are good source of iron which regenerates and reactivates the red blood cells and supplies fresh oxygen to the body. The copper content in beets helps make the iron more available to the body.

Anxiety

Anxiety causes a general state of worry, fear, nervousness, fear and apprehension. Anxiety affects how we feel and behave, and can even manifest in physical symptoms. Certain foods can help you overcome mild to moderate anxiety.

Peanuts

Gamma aminobutyric acid (GABA) is an atypical amino acid that acts as a neurotransmitter in your central nervous system. It has a calming effect and helps to reduce anxiety and nervousness. If you're not producing enough GABA, you are likely to feel anxious and nervous. Peanuts are one of the best sources of glutamine, the amino acid needed to make GABA.

Arteriosclerosis

Arteriosclerosis, or hardening of the arteries, occurs when too much pressure in the arteries make the walls thick and stiff and restrict blood flow to the organs and tissues.

Beets

The juice of this wonderful root is a powerful solvent for inorganic calcium deposits that cause the arteries to harden and therefore it is very useful in fighting arteriosclerosis. It helps to keep the blood vessels and the arterial system in a very sound condition.

Asthma Inflammation

Asthma is a chronic inflammatory lung disease that causes wheezing, difficulty breathing and chest tightness. Medications and foods aimed at reducing inflammation play a major role in treating and managing asthma. Eating foods that reduce inflammation can help you better control your asthma.

Carrots

Carrots are a top source for beta-carotene, hence the name. Beta-carotene may reduce lung inflammation caused by toxins and may also decrease asthma symptoms caused by exercise.

Oranges

Asthma symptoms can be triggered by allergens, such as pollen or pet dander and by non-allergic triggers, such as emotional stress, physical activity, cold air, smoke, or viruses. Consuming oranges and other citrus fruits may help reduce your symptoms. Citrus fruits are rich sources of vitamin A and C which help lessen lung inflammation associated with cigarette smoke and other pollutants.

Pineapple

The bromelain in pineapple has been shown to reduce asthma inflammation. Studies have found that bromelain can significantly reduce markers of lung inflammation and reduce the total white blood cells which normally increase with the onset of asthma.

Warning: While some foods can be beneficial for asthma inflammation, it is important to remember that not all treatments work the same for everyone. Asthma attacks can be life threatening; for your own safety, please speak to your doctor before initiating any alternative asthma therapy and/or discontinuing your use of prescription medications.

Bone Loss

Bones are living tissues, like muscle, which respond to diet and exercise. Bone loss occurs when bones are broken down faster than they are being made. Bone loss can lead to low bone density and eventually osteoporosis.

Dairy Products

It is of course no secret that milk and other dairy products are one of the best sources of calcium and vitamin D, both of which are needed for healthy bones. If you can't consume dairy products due to lactose intolerance or food allergies, there are other good sources of calcium such as tofu, calcium fortified juices and soy milk.

Green Leafy Vegetables

Green leafy vegetables are high in vitamin K which is critical in forming bone proteins and reducing calcium loss. Vitamin K has been shown to not only increase bone density in people with osteoporosis, but also reduce fracture rates. One cup of cooked collards contains more than 25% of your daily calcium.

Olives

Hydroxytyrosol is a phytonutrient in olive oil that has been found to have the potential to help us prevent bone loss. Several studies have found increased depositing of calcium in bone and decreased loss of total bone mass following consumption of this olive phytonutrient.

Brain Fog

Brain fog or mental fog, is a term used to describe the subjective sensation of mental clouding described as feeling "foggy." Brain fog can include forgetfulness, difficulty recalling known words, easily becoming lost, confusion, trouble concentrating, and just a general sense of slow foggy thinking. For many people, brain fog can be severe and can have a big an impact on their lives.

Apple

Eating apples can improve your memory and help you sustain overall brain health. Apples contain a larger percentage of phosphorus than any other fruit or vegetable. For this reason it is an invaluable food for brain health. The effects of the antioxidants and flavonoids present in apples have been shown to reduce brain-cell inflammation and oxidation that occurs naturally due to the presence of free radicals. Eating apples increases acetylcholine, which is a critical neurotransmitter for memory and brain health. Sufferers from cognitive problems such as brain fog and poor memory should eat at least two apples every day.

Cancer

Cancer is a leading cause of death around the world. Nutrition can be an important part of cancer prevention and treatment. Nutrition is a low cost therapy that can help to prevent or significantly delay the onset of many types of cancers and also substantially improve the quality and quantity of life for medically treated cancer patients. The right foods can help to change the underlying causes of cancer, thus paving the way for long term favorable outcome in cancer treatment.

Asparagus

Asparagus is packed with antioxidants which help neutralize cell-damaging free radicals. Asparagus is the best food source of glutathione, a detoxifying compound that helps break down carcinogens and other harmful compounds. In addition, Asparin A, a compound in asparagus, has been found to halt the growth liver cancer cells and can even cause death in those cells. Chronic inflammation and oxidative stress are risk factors for a variety of cancer types. The steroidal glycosides compounds in asparagus have strong anti-inflammatory and antioxidant properties.

Blackberries

Blackberries are particularly rich in anthocyanins, which have antioxidant and anti-inflammatory properties. According to a study published *The Journal of Biological Chemistry,* the anthocyanins in blackberries may help prevent or inhibit the growth of cancerous cells. In addition, the high concentration of antioxidants found in blackberries may help prevent free radical damage, thereby reducing the risk of chronic conditions such as cancer.

Blueberries

Blueberries contain phenolic compounds which, in harmony with anthocyanin and other antioxidants, can do wonders to prevent or treat cancers. Studies published in the *Journal of Agricultural and Food Chemistry* showed that the phenolic compounds in blueberries can inhibit colon cancer cell proliferation. Another study at the Beckman Research Institute showed that blueberries have the potential to inhibit the growth of Triple Negative Breast Cancer, a particularly aggressive form of breast tumor.

Broccoli

Diets high in broccoli have been linked with a lower risk of certain types of cancer. Broccoli contains certain chemicals that work through numerous mechanisms to inhibit tumor cell adhesion, spread, and invasion. These substances act as antioxidants, boost detoxifying enzymes in the body, and may even produce beneficial changes in gene expression. Studies suggest that a broccoli compound known as sulforaphane induces cancer cells to commit a sort of cellular suicide.

Garlic

Several studies have shown a link between increased garlic intake and reduced risk of certain cancers, including cancers of the stomach, colon, esophagus, pancreas, and breast. Another study showed that women who ate the most garlic had a 50% lower risk of cancer of the colon compared with women who ate the least.

Grapefruit

Pink and red grapefruits are excellent sources of lycopene. Lycopene has a high capacity to help fight oxygen free radicals and is a powerful agent against tumors and cancers. Grapefruit also contains liminoids and naringenin. Liminoids may help prevent cancerous cells from proliferating and also inhibit tumor formation by promoting the formation of glutathione-S-transferase, a detoxifying enzyme. Naringenin is an antioxidant compound which has been shown to repair damaged DNA in prostate cancer cells.

Mangoes

Mangoes are rich in phenols, such as quercetin, isoquercitrin, astragalin, fisetin, gallic acid and methylgallat, and enzymes which have cancer preventing capacities. Mangoes are also high in a soluble fiber which has been linked to a lower risk of cancers of the gastrointestinal tract. Mangoes also provide vitamin C which helps protect cells from free radical damage and reduces the risk of cancer.

Olives

Olives are a great source of vitamin E and monounsaturated fat, which have the ability to neutralize free radicals in the body. If our cells get overwhelmed by oxidative stress caused by free radicals and chronic excessive inflammation, our risk of cancer is increased. By providing us with rich supplies of antioxidant and anti-inflammatory nutrients, olives can help us avoid this dangerous combination of chronic oxidative stress and chronic inflammation.

Studies have shown that olive oil exerts a protective effect against certain malignant tumors in the breast, prostate, and digestive tract. Olive oil rich diets have been shown to reduce the number of cancerous lesions, result in less aggressive tumors and a better prognosis.

Papaya

Papaya can be very beneficial for reducing your risk of developing certain types of cancers. Studies suggest that the proteolytic enzymes in papaya can digest the fibrin protein layer of cancer cells that usually surrounds and protects them, leaving the cancerous cells more susceptible to the body's immune response. Papayas also contain isothiocyanates which may help prevent cancer by eliminating potential carcinogens from our bodies and enhancing the action of tumor suppressing proteins and lycopene, which research has shown to have anticancer properties.

Tomato

Tomatoes are a natural cancer fighter. Lycopene is rare in foods, and tomatoes are one of only a few foods that are naturally rich in this powerful antioxidant. Clinical studies have shown that lycopene can reduce the risk of cancers such as prostate, cervical, mouth, throat, stomach, colon, rectal, prostate, and ovarian cancer. In addition, the vitamin A and C in tomatoes fight the free radicals which can cause cell damage. Ironically, processed tomatoes (sauce, paste, etc.) are more effective than raw tomatoes at reducing cancer risk. The processing breaks down the cell walls which trap the lycopene making it more bioavailable. Tomatoes have been shown to be particularly effective against prostate cancers.

Candidiasis

Candidiasis is a yeast infection caused by an overgrowth of the bacterial yeast Candida Albicans. It can manifest as a vaginal yeast infection, oral thrush, jock itch, or diaper rash. We all have some amount of yeast on our skin and in our bodies, but when an overgrowth of yeast occurs, we can experience very unpleasant symptoms; this is referred to as a yeast infection or candidiasis. The

Candida yeast feeds on sugar and multiplies very quickly.

Garlic and Yogurt

The best way to combat the overgrowth of Candida yeast is to simultaneously starve it, by eliminating sugar from your diet, and repopulate the good bacteria in your body through the use of probiotics and antibacterial substances such as yogurt and garlic. Treatment combining the antibacterial and antifungal actions of garlic with the probiotic effects of yogurt can be very effective against candidiasis.

Canker Sore

Canker sores can be quite uncomfortable or even painful. Canker sores should not be confused with cold sores. Cold sores or fever blisters are caused by a virus and typically appear outside of the mouth. Canker sores, on the other hand, are small ulcers that appear inside of the mouth and can make eating and talking quite uncomfortable. Canker sores may be small, but they can be hard to ignore. Fortunately, a canker sore is generally pretty short-lived, and there are home remedies you can use to get some temporary relief.

Lemons

Lemons have antibacterial which can accelerate the healing process of canker sores. Mix the juice of freshly squeezed lemon into a glass of lukewarm water and rinse your mouth with this solution several times a day.

Chest Congestion

Chest congestion occurs when excess fluid and mucus accumulate in the lungs. Severe chest congestion can lead to more serious health issues like pneumonia or bronchitis. You should do all you can to relieve and clear up a congested chest before it worsens.

Orange

Chest congestion can make breathing difficult and can cause coughing and shortness of breath. Oranges have an effect on the secretion of mucus by the glands lining your respiratory system. Oranges are also rich in vitamin C which is an essential nutrient that may help increase the effectiveness of your immune system. This can help reduce the severity and duration of conditions that cause chest congestion. Oranges are also a natural source of water, which can help reduce the thickness of mucus.

Chronic Inflammation

Inflammation is the body's response to harmful stimuli, such as pathogens, damaged cells, or irritants. It is an attempt at removing the harmful stimuli from the body and begin the healing process. Chronic inflammation can lead to a host of diseases. It can lead to serious metabolic breakdown with serious implications for your long-term health.

Blackberries

Inflammation is really the cause of a lot of our ill health. As we age, we become more susceptible to free radical damage and inflammation. Blackberries are full of antioxidants which protect the body against inflammation and free radicals. More specifically, studies have shown that the phenolic components of blackberries exhibit powerful anti-inflammatory properties and inhibit the activity of inflammatory chemicals such as interleukins.

Blueberries

Blueberries are excellent anti-inflammatories and pain relievers. Blueberries increase the amounts of compounds called heat-shock proteins which help reduce inflammation and pain. Blueberries also contain salicylic acid which is the natural version of aspirin and is known to thin the blood and reduce pain.

Olive Oil

The monounsaturated fats, vitamin E, and polyphenols in olive oil have anti-inflammatory abilities. Olive oil also contains a chemical called oleocanthal, which acts as a painkiller and inhibits inflammation by the same means that drugs like Ibuprofen do.

Circulation Problems

Blood circulation is responsible for moving oxygen, nutrients and wastes to and from our organs and cells. It also helps stabilize body temperature and pH to maintain harmony. When circulation is compromised, oxygen does not reach all of the organs.

Beets

Beet juice is best known as a blood purifier and blood builder that help in the creation of red blood cells. Beet juice can help in the construction of red blood cells which help to carry oxygen around the body. Beets contain nitrate which causes dilation of the blood cells allowing more blood to get around the veins thereby reducing high blood pressure. This then improves circulation.

Constipation

No one likes talking about constipation. Constipation can be a painful and frustrating problem. People who are constipated may find it difficult and painful to have a bowel movement. Constipation is often the result of low fiber diets. Simply adding more fiber can be an effective remedy.

Brazil Nut

Adding brazil nuts to your diet may provide much needed relief. Brazil nuts are high in selenium and fiber which help get things moving.

Flaxseed

Flax seed are high in fiber. You'd be hard-pressed to find a food higher in fiber than flax

Cough

Coughing is the body's way of ridding itself of mucus from the lungs, or of reacting to an irritated airway. A coughing fit can be very frustrating, especially when you are trying to sleep.

Thyme

The next time you have a cold or cough, try a cup of thyme tea. Thyme has been shown to have bronchodilating and antispasmodic effects, so it helps to relax the bronchial tubes and alleviates coughing fits. Thyme oil is used in many cough syrups because it acts as an expectorant loosening mucous and has antibacterial and antiseptic properties.

Depression

Depression is complex disease which can occur for a variety of reasons. People that experience depression may feel overwhelmed with sadness and loneliness for no known reason. Many antidepressants act by inhibiting the reuptake of serotonin by receptors in the brain, therefore increasing serotonin levels. If you are experiencing mild to moderate depression, you may be able to increase your brain's serotonin levels by eating foods that boost your serotonin levels naturally.

Beets

Depression has been linked with lower levels of folate. One cup of beets supplies you with 30% of your daily needs. Beets contain trimethylglycine, the same substance that is used in certain treatments of depression. It also contains tryptophan, which relaxes the mind and creates a sense of well-being.

Cacao (Chocolate)

Cacao is a mood enhancer. Phenylethylamine, in combination with theobromine, can elevate mood and create a sense well-being. Eating cacao can raise your natural levels of serotonin and create a balancing effect.

Diarrhea

Diarrhea is uncomfortable, unpleasant and possibly embarrassing. Fortunately, the vast majority of diarrhea cases are simple and short lived. Gastroenteritis is one of the most common causes of diarrhea. Eating or drinking foods contaminated with bacteria can also cause diarrhea. There are certain foods that can help ease your symptoms.

Blackberries

Blackberries are one of the best foods around for the treatment of diarrhea. Blackberries contain tannins that help to tone the intestinal tract and soothe diarrhea. They also help prevent the irritating and toxic substances that cause diarrhea from being absorbed back into the bloodstream.

Dull Hair

Spinach

Spinach is excellent for overall hair health and shine. Spinach is loaded with vitamins A and C, which help your body to create sebum, the oil secreted by follicles to give your hair gloss and shine.

Erectile Dysfunction

Erectile dysfunction (ED) is the inability to achieve or sustain an erection. Problems getting an erection can be very stressful, cause relationship problems or affect a man's self-confidence. Erectile dysfunction can be a sign of a bigger health condition such as heart disease or diabetes. Although there's no miracle food to prevent erectile dysfunction, evidence suggests that certain foods may help by addressing the underlying problem.

Beets

Some foods increase circulation because of their high concentration of nitrates. Beets contain a high amount of nitrate which causes dilation of the blood cells allowing more blood to get around the veins. Nitrates have been shown to have beneficial effects for erectile dysfunction. Prescription ED medications are based on the relaxing effects of nitrates on the blood vessels that supply the penis.

Garlic

In order to maintain an erection, the arteries need to have an efficient blood flow. Crushed garlic contains allicin, a compound that can decrease blood pressure and improve blood flow, which may lead to a harder erection.

Gas and Bloating

Everyone has gas. Gas and bloating doesn't necessarily mean there is something wrong with your digestion, but excessive gas can be uncomfortable and embarrassing. There are foods that can help minimize embarrassing gas.

Thyme

Thyme is often recommended to promote good digestion and relieve gas and bloating. The volatile oils in thyme help reduce gas while its phenols work as an antispasmodic, helping to relieve intestinal cramping.

Gastritis

Gastritis is an inflammation of the lining of the stomach. The most common symptoms are upset stomach, pain, indigestion, abdominal bloating, nausea, and vomiting. There are certain foods that can provide some symptom relief.

Banana

Bananas are a good choice to settle an upset digestive system. Bananas normalize colonic functions in the large intestine by absorbing large amounts of water. The high level of potassium in bananas helps to replace electrolytes that may be lost during bouts of diarrhea. Bananas contain insoluble fiber, which helps relieve constipation.

They also contain inulin, a prebiotic soluble fiber that promotes the growth of beneficial bacteria in the intestinal system.

Papaya

Undigested proteins can lead to many health issues, such as gastrointestinal problems and an overgrowth of flatulence causing bacteria in the colon. The primary therapeutic enzyme in papayas, papain, is a cysteine protease enzyme that is well known for its various digestive health benefits. Papayas improve digestion by breaking down proteins into their individual amino acids and dissolving fats. Its anti-inflammatory effects also help to soothe upset stomach.

Pineapple

Suffering from gastrointestinal or digestive problems is not fun. Pineapples are one of the best foods to help promote healthy digestion and ease gastrointestinal problems. Pineapples can help us avoid digestive problems like gas, bloating, upset stomach, diarrhea, burping and constipation. The bromelain in pineapple improves digestion by breaking down hard to digest proteins into their individual amino acids. Pineapples are also rich in fiber which offers additional digestive benefits.

Gout

Gout occurs when the body has high levels of uric acid and is characterized by recurrent attacks of acute inflammatory arthritis. Gout symptoms occur when excess uric acid forms sharp crystals which collect between the joints and cause painful inflammation.

Apples

The malic acid contained in apples helps to neutralize uric acid. Daily consumption of apples can help reduce gout attacks.

Halitosis (Bad Breath)

Halitosis is very personal and often embarrassing problems commonly faced by millions of people.

Lemons

Although lemons might be mouth-puckering to the taste, the citric acid in lemons can help to neutralize bad-breath smells. Chewing on fresh lemons or rinsing with lemon juice can help freshen breath after consuming certain foods, spices, alcohol, or cigarettes.

Parsley

Bad breath can be an embarrassing nuisance especially in social situations. Parsley contains chemicals that help to freshen bad breath. Parsley is rich in chlorophyll which has antioxidant and anti-inflammatory properties and helps to neutralize toxins and pollutants and act as a natural deodorizer. Chewing a small handful of parsley allows you to gain the breath-freshening benefits of chlorophyll. This may be reason why parsley makes an appearance as a garnish on so many restaurant dishes.

Heart Disease

Heart disease is a leading cause of death. Although you cannot control certain factors like age and family history, you can use food and nutrition to help you prevent heart disease.

Apples

Apples are full of antioxidant compounds which help inhibit inflammation and lower levels of cholesterol and two other markers associated with plaque and inflammation in artery walls. Apples are also high in fiber which has been shown to lower cholesterol level. Studies have shown that frequent apple eaters have reduced risk of suffering from heart attacks and strokes compared with non-apple eaters.

Blackberries

Blackberries may help to prevent heart disease by inactivating the enzymes that damage the endothelial cells lining the blood vessels. They contain high amounts of fiber, are rich in polyphenols, vitamin C, and contain a bit of iron, calcium, and vitamin A. The antioxidants in blackberries also protect the cells of the cardiovascular system from harmful effects of unstable oxygen radicals.

Blueberries

Blueberries have a high anthocyanin content. Anthocyanin has been shown to dilate arteries, counter the buildup of plaque, and provide other cardiovascular benefits. Blueberries are also rich in fiber and antioxidants which also help reduce the likelihood of heart attacks. A Harvard School of Public Health study published in the January 2013 issue of the *Journal of the American Heart Association,* found that eating three or more servings of blueberries per week may reduce a woman's risk of heart attack by as much as 33%.

Carrots

Diets high in carrots are associated with a lower risk of heart disease. Carrots are high in fiber and beta-carotene, nutrients which help keep blood pressure down and reduce cholesterol levels, thus reducing the risk of heart disease. Studies indicate that consuming about 2 baby carrots daily can lower the risk of coronary heart disease by approximately 32%.

Coconut

Many people can't imagine how a food high in saturated fat, like coconut, can be beneficial for the heart. Coconut oil is beneficial for the heart because it contains about 50% lauric acid, which helps in preventing various heart problems including high cholesterol levels and high blood pressure. In addition, the saturated fats present in coconut oil are Medium Chain Triglycerides (MCT's) which do not lead to an increase in LDL levels. Coconut actually protects against heart disease by increasing good cholesterol and lowering the ratio of bad to good cholesterol.

Kiwi

Kiwi can be considered a superfood for your heart. The Cleveland Clinic has recommended kiwis as one of the most powerful foods for the heart. Kiwis help to lower triglyceride levels and reduce platelet hyperactivity which plays a role in the development and stability of atherosclerotic vascular plaques and limits the tendency of blood to form clots. The vitamin C and E in kiwis, combined with the polyphenols and magnesium, potassium, B vitamins, and copper, act to protect the cardiovascular system.

Hot Peppers

Hot peppers are a heart healthy food. The compounds in hot peppers, including capsaicin, have been found to lower blood pressure, decrease cholesterol levels, and reduce the risk for dangerous blood clots.

Oats

The accumulation of cholesterol is implicated in many types of cardiovascular disease. Oatmeal and oat bran are significant sources of soluble and insoluble fiber. One component of the soluble fiber found in oats is beta-glucans, which has proven effective in lowering blood cholesterol. Oats are also one of the best sources of compounds called tocotrienols which inhibit cholesterol synthesis and have been found to lower blood cholesterol.

Research also indicates that the antioxidants found in oats reduce cholesterol by reducing the ability of blood cells to stick to the inside of artery walls. A daily bowl of oatmeal can lower cholesterol by up to 23 percent and reduce the risk of heart disease by almost half.

Olives

Oleuropein is found exclusively in olives and has been shown to decrease oxidation of LDL cholesterol. In addition, the high monounsaturated fat content of olives has been associated with reduced risk of cardiovascular disease and decreased blood pressure. The oleic acid found in olives affects changes at cell membrane levels which result in decreased blood pressure.

Pomegranate

The potent antioxidant compounds in pomegranates have been shown to reduce platelet aggregation, reduce atherosclerosis, and lower blood pressure. A recent medical study published in the journal of *Clinical Nutrition* found that patients with severe carotid artery blockages who drank a glass a pomegranate juice every day for a year saw a 12% reduction in blood pressure and a 30% reduction in atherosclerotic plaque.

Pomegranates contain high levels of flavonoids and polyphenols, potent antioxidants that protect against heart disease.

High Blood Pressure

High blood pressure is a chronic condition in which the pressure of the blood against the artery walls is elevated. This requires the heart to work harder than normal to circulate blood through the blood vessels. High blood pressure increases the risk for heart disease and strokes. You can make dietary changes that will help keep your blood pressure levels normal.

Broccoli

Research indicates that glucoraphanin, a compound found in broccoli, may reduce the risk of high blood pressure. Broccoli also contains potassium, magnesium, and calcium which also help regulate blood pressure.

Spinach

Spinach is low in calories, high in fiber, and packed with heart-healthy nutrients like potassium, folate, and magnesium. Spinach contains almost 40% of magnesium your body needs. Magnesium is essential in maintaining healthy levels of blood pressure. In fact, just a salad-size portion of spinach will work to lower high blood pressure within hours.

High Blood Sugar

High blood sugar happens when your body makes too little insulin or when your body is not able to use insulin properly. Insulin helps the body use glucose for energy. High levels of sugar in the blood can be harmful. There are foods that can help you keep your blood sugar levels low.

Artichoke

An artichoke has a glycemic index ranking of 15, which places it among the very lowest foods or beverages on the glycemic index. Scientific evidence shows that the artichoke can help balance blood glucose levels. Glycogen is stored in the body and turned into sugar whenever blood sugar supplies are low. The overproduction of glucose by the liver can lead to diabetes and other health problems. The cynarin present in artichokes can keep the liver from producing too much glucose.

Cinnamon

Cinnamon has been shown to be of great value in maintaining healthy blood sugar levels. Cinnamon mimics the effects of insulin and has a regulatory effect on blood sugar, making it especially beneficial for people with Type 2 diabetes. The American Diabetes Association has found that taking 3 to 6 grams of cinnamon per day can lower glucose levels in people with Type 2 diabetes. A recent study published in the *American Journal of Clinical Nutrition* found that consuming about teaspoon of cinnamon even helped tame blood sugar in people without diabetes.

High Cholesterol

Cholesterol is a waxy fat-like substance which is an essential part of cells in the body. Cholesterol is so important to our bodies, that the body can actually make all of the cholesterol it needs; however, most of us also get cholesterol from our diet. When there is too much LDL cholesterol in the blood, it forms deposits or plaques in the artery walls which narrow the arteries and limit blood flow. Heart attacks and strokes are caused when this plaque breaks apart. Keeping our levels of total and LDL cholesterols low is very important to our health. A healthy diet can go a long way towards reducing high cholesterol levels.

Avocado

The oleic acid in avocados can help lower total cholesterol and LDL cholesterol levels while increasing the HDL (good cholesterol) levels. Avocados are also rich in fiber and beta-sitosterol, both of which help keep cholesterol levels low.

Almonds

Almonds are rich in dietary fiber, vitamins, and minerals, and are packed with numerous health promoting phytochemicals. Almonds contain unsaturated fatty acids like oleic and palmitoleic acids which have been shown to lower blood LDL (bad cholesterol) and increase HDL (good cholesterol) levels thus helping to prevent coronary artery disease and strokes.

Cinnamon

Cinnamon contains polyphenols which create healthier arteries and reduce the risk of cardiovascular disease. Scientists have found evidence that cinnamon helps lower lipid levels. Just ½ teaspoon of cinnamon per day may help you lower triglycerides and LDL cholesterol levels.

Grapefruit

Grapefruits can help reduce cholesterol levels. Grapefruits are high in antioxidants and contain pectin, a soluble fiber that has been shown to slow down the progression of atherosclerosis. Studies have shown that grapefruits can reduce blood levels of LDL cholesterol and triglycerides. Both red and blond grapefruits can positively influence cholesterol levels, but red grapefruit is more effective, especially in lowering triglycerides.

Mango

Mangoes have high levels of soluble fiber, pectin and vitamin C, all of which help to lower serum cholesterol levels, especially LDL cholesterol (the bad cholesterol). Research suggests that compounds in mangoes could ease the effects of high cholesterol.

IBS

The cause of IBS is still not yet clear; what is clear is that IBS can be very painful and uncomfortable and that certain foods can cause flare ups. The most common triggers foods are dairy products, wheat (gluten), sweeteners, beans, carbonated beverages and alcohol. It is not only important to know what trigger foods to avoid, but also what foods can help your symptoms.

Coconut

Extra virgin coconut oil has been shown to help improve the digestive system and thus prevents various stomach and digestion related problems including irritable bowel syndrome. The saturated fats present in coconut oil have antimicrobial properties which can help control the bacteria, fungi and parasites that cause indigestion and irritable bowel symptoms.

Kidney Stones

If you've ever passed a kidney stone, you won't forget the sudden, intense pain. Kidney stones form when urine in the kidney becomes supersaturated with stone-forming salts.

Lemon

Lemon juice increases the amount of citrate in the urine which helps to inhibit kidney stones from forming. If you are prone to kidney stones, you may want to consider drinking low sugar or sugar-free lemonade on a regular basis. Scientific evidence suggests that drinking 1 to 2 liters of lemon juice as lemonade per day can help you lower the risk of developing kidney stones.

Liver Ailments

The liver is one of the most important organs of the body. Your liver plays a vital role in your health and vitality. Having a healthy liver results in greater energy and general sense of well-being. A poorly functioning liver can result in tiredness, headaches, allergies, problem skin and weight gain.

Apple

Apples contain pectin which keeps the liver from absorbing cholesterol and binds to heavy metals in the body (in particular in the colon) to help their excretion. This reduces the load on the liver and its detoxification capacities. The malic acid in apples also helps to break up gall stones.

Artichoke

Few veggies are as potent as the artichoke in helping an ailing liver. Studies have found they may even regenerate liver tissue. Experts believe that artichokes help stimulate production of bile in the liver as well as promote the movement of bile through the system. These two functions are vital to the liver's well-being. One of the jobs of bile is to remove toxins through the bowel. If bile is not transported adequately, the liver has an increased risk of being damaged. It has been suggested that 30 minutes after eating globe artichoke, bile flow is increased by over 100%. Artichokes have long been used in folk and alternative medicine as a treatment for liver ailments and the scientific studies are now proving them to be correct.

Broccoli

The liver is one of the most important organs of the body. It is responsible for regulating blood sugar, absorbing nutrients, and eliminating harmful substances from the body. Broccoli is a very powerful detoxifier of the liver. Broccoli increases the amount of glucosinolate which help the liver to produce the enzymes it needs for its detoxification processes. Broccoli also contains chemicals that neutralize certain toxins.

Garlic

Garlic contains allicin which is a sulphur-based compound needed by the liver for effective detoxification. The antioxidants in garlic help keep toxic substances filtered by your liver from reaching other organs. Garlic has been shown to help the liver rid the body of mercury, food additives, and the hormone estrogen.

Low Sex Drive

There are various types of foods you can try to help increase your sex drive and fight impotence, and most of the fruits that help to increase your sex drive will contain high levels of certain vitamins on minerals which may help to increase hormone levels, increase nitric oxide levels or ramp up your testosterone.

Mango

Mangoes are rich in vitamins C and E. Vitamin E has been proven to regulate sex hormones and boost sex drive. Research conducted at the University of Maryland Medical Center suggests that vitamin C can help with sexual problems such erectile dysfunction and a low libido.

Pomegranate

Pomegranates have been shown to increase low sex drive. Studies indicate that drinking pomegranate juice daily for 2 weeks can elevate levels of sexual interest in both men and women by increasing their levels of testosterone. Pomegranates also help the body produce nitric oxide which helps to open up blood vessels and increase to blood flow which in turns increases libido.

Macular Degeneration

Macular degeneration is a chronic eye disease that causes vision loss marked by degeneration of the macula in the center of retina. Macular degeneration affects our ability to see fine detail and sharp images. Macular degeneration has no cure, but nutrition can be used to help prevent or slow the progression of the disease.

Blueberries

Blueberries have the potential to slow down visual loss and prevent or delay age related ocular problems like macular degeneration and cataract due to their high levels of antioxidants including carotenoids (lutein, zeaxanthin), flavonoids (resveritrol, quercetin), vitamin C, vitamins E and A, selenium, zinc and phosphorus.

Carrots

Carrots are rich in beta-carotene and lutein which are vital for eye health. Beta-carotene is an important precursor for vitamin A. Severe deficiencies in vitamin A can cause blindness. Beta-carotene helps to protect against macular degeneration and the development of senile cataracts. Studies have found that people who eat the plenty of carrots have a much lower risk of macular degeneration than those who eat very little.

Tomato

The vitamin A that tomatoes provide can improve vision and help prevent eye conditions such as night blindness and macular degeneration. A deficiency in vitamin A contributes to the development of night blindness. A one cup serving of fresh tomatoes provides 30% of the daily value of vitamin A.

Meniere's Disease

Meniere's disease is an idiopathic disease involving the inner ear that is characterized by vertigo, hearing loss and pain, nausea and tinnitus.

Lemon

Meniere's disease does not have a cure; however lemons may bring some relief to those who suffer from this disease. Research has shown that Meniere's disease patients treated with lemon bioflavonoid complex saw improvements in their vertigo and hearing symptoms. Although the exact physiologic mechanism by which this effect is produced is unknown, it is hypothesized that the bioflavonoids in lemon may act as a blocking agent on histidine decarboxylase.

Muscle Cramps

Muscle cramps are a common problem and can be very painful. They are often caused by straining or overusing a muscle, mineral depletion, dehydration, or not enough blood reading the muscles.

Bananas

A deficiency in potassium can cause muscle cramps and spasms, as well as greater susceptibility to injury. Bananas are high in potassium and thus can help relieve muscle cramps and spasms.

Cherries

Post-workout muscle soreness can be quite a pain. If you're looking for a healthy way to ease post-exercise soreness, cherries might be a great option. Cherries contain the same anti-inflammatory enzymes as Ibuprofen, without the potential side effects. Cherries contain high levels of polyphenols, which reduce inflammation, tenderness and pain.

Night Blindness

Night Blindness is a condition that makes it difficult to see in relatively low light. Night blindness is not a disorder itself, but rather a symptom of other diseases of the eye.

Tomatoes

The vitamin A that tomatoes provide can improve vision and help prevent night blindness. A deficiency in vitamin A contributes to the development of night blindness. A one cup serving of fresh tomatoes provides 30% of the daily value of vitamin A.

Osteoporosis

Osteoporosis is a disease in which bones have become weak, porous and fragile. Porous bones are more likely to break. Osteoporosis is a serious disease that affects millions of people worldwide. Without prevention or treatment, osteoporosis can progress until a bone fractures. Fractures commonly occur in the hip, spine, and wrist.

Dairy Products

Milk and other dairy products are one of the best sources of calcium and vitamin D, both of which are needed for healthy bones.

Olives

Hydroxytyrosol is a phytonutrient in olive oil has been found to have the potential to help prevent bone loss. Several studies have found increased depositing of calcium in bone and decreased loss of total bone mass following consumption of this olive phytonutrient.

Pumpkin Seeds

Magnesium and calcium work together to promote bone health. 50% of the body's magnesium resides in the bones and low levels have been linked to fragile bones. Pumpkin seeds are an excellent source of magnesium.

Tomato

Tomatoes build strong bones and can ward off osteoporosis. Lycopene slows down the breakdown of bone cells and the vitamin K and calcium in tomatoes help strengthen and repair bones. A serving of tomatoes provides 18% the daily value for vitamin K.

Spinach

One cup of cooked spinach provides over 1000% of the daily recommended vitamin K which helps prevent excess activation of osteoclasts, the cells that break down bones. Vitamin K also promotes the synthesis of osteocalcin, an essential protein for maintaining the strength and density of our bones.

Pain

Chronic inflammation contributes to many painful conditions, including back pain and arthritis. Over-the-counter anti-inflammatory medications such as Ibuprofen tend to work well but can have their own side effects such as stomach upset.

Blueberries

Blueberries are excellent anti-inflammatories and pain relievers. Blueberries increase the amounts of compounds called heat-shock proteins which help reduce inflammation and pain. Blueberries also contain salicylic acid which is the natural version of aspirin and is known to thin the blood and reduce pain.

Hot Peppers

Capsaicin, the active ingredient in hot peppers, has been shown to reduce pain. It acts by binding to receptors in the cell wall of nerve endings and triggering an influx of calcium ions into the neurons. It also interferes with substance P, a chemical involved in transmitting pain impulses to the brain.

Poor Circulation

Poor circulation is when blood flow becomes restricted to certain parts of the body such as the toes and fingers. Poor circulation can cause a lot of discomfort and can lead to more serious health problems. There are foods that can help you improve your circulation.

Beets

Beet juice is best known as a blood purifier and blood builder that help in the creation of red blood cells. Beet juice can help in the construction of red blood cells which help to carry oxygen around the body. Beets contain nitrate which causes dilation of the blood cells allowing more blood to get around the veins thereby reducing high blood pressure. This then improves circulation.

Respiratory Problems

Your lungs are constantly bombarded by toxins, such as air pollution, cigarette smoke and allergens. This exposure can lead to lung cancer, bronchitis and other respiratory ailments.

Kiwis

This nutrient dense fruit pack more vitamin C than oranges and is especially effective against respiratory problems such as shortness of breath, asthma and cough. Studies indicate that kiwi eaters are less likely to experience wheezing, shortness of breath, or runny noses.

Restless Leg Syndrome

Those who experience restless leg syndrome have difficulty getting a good night's sleep because they are seized by uncontrollable urge to move their leg while in bed. Because RLS often results in sleep deprivation, it can lead to anxiety and depression.

Spinach

Restless Leg Syndrome has been associated with low levels of iron, magnesium and folate. Foods high in these nutrients have been shown to be helpful in easing the symptoms of RLS. Spinach, along with other green leafy vegetables like mustard greens and kale, are rich in folate, iron, and magnesium.

Sinus Infections

Infections occur when foreign organisms gets into a person's body and cause harm. There are many kinds of infection causing agents including viruses, bacteria, parasites, and fungus. Sinus infections are generally a bacterial infection. Sinus infections can be very painful and uncomfortable.

Garlic

Garlic has been shown to be quite effective at treating sinus infections. Garlic contains allicin which is a powerful antibiotic and a potent agent that helps the body to inhibit the ability of germs to grow and reproduce. Garlic has been used effectively against a whole host of bacteria, fungus, and viruses. Some studies suggest that garlic is an even more powerful bacteria-killer than either penicillin or tetracycline.

Skin Problems

Many skin conditions can be managed or improved by using food and nutrition.

Mango

If you suffer from skin problems, you may want to think about adding mangoes to your diet. Applying mangoes directly to the skin will help to get rid of clogged pores, however eating mangoes regularly helps to reduce dry skin and flakiness, leaving the skin soft and shining from the inside out.

Lemon

Lemons have healing properties that work well to heal skin blemishes. Applied externally, lemons decrease inflammation, redness and irritation from acne and restore skin to health. Lemons are rich in vitamin C which has anti-inflammatory properties and alpha-hydroxy acid which works as a skin exfoliator.

Sleep Problems

Nothing is worse than suffering from insomnia or poor sleep. Not only is it frustrating, but research poor sleep can be detrimental to our health.

Cherries

The antioxidant melatonin significantly improves the body's sleep pattern and sleep quality. Cherries are one of the few foods that contain melatonin. Cherries can increase melatonin levels in the blood, therefore improving the way you sleep. A cup of tart cherries or glass of tart cherry juice can improve the duration and quality of your sleep.

Sore Throat

An inflamed sore throat can be difficult to cope with. Sore throats are often caused by allergies, bacterial infections or viral infections including the common cold. Sore throats are often accompanied fever, chills, swollen lymph nodes, and pain while swallowing.

Lemon and Honey

A mixture of lemon and honey makes an excellent sore throat relieving alternative. Honey has been proven effective against many kinds of bacteria and lemons enhance the antimicrobial properties of the honey. Lemons are also high in vitamin C which boosts the immune system. Lemons also work to reduce inflammation and thin mucous congestion.

Urinary Tract Infection

Urinary tract infection (UTI) is caused when bacteria gets into the urinary tract (urethra, bladder, ureters and kidneys) causing an infection. The bladder and urethra are most commonly affected by UTI's. If you've ever suffered from a UTI, you most likely experienced painful, burning urination, exhaustion and discomfort.

Blueberries

Everybody knows that cranberries help fight urinary tract infections, but for those of us who do not appreciate their tartness, blueberries are an excellent choice. Blueberries have been shown to be quite beneficial to urinary tract health. Bacteria like b-coli are responsible for urinary tract infections. Blueberries have a compound which inhibits the growth of these bacteria. Blueberries also have some antibiotic properties which add to this effect.

Weight Problems

There are of course foods that promote weight gain and foods that promote weight loss. We all know the common culprits that drive weight gain (fried foods, sugar, sweetened beverages, processed meats, and starchy carbs) but here are some of the best foods to help you lose or maintain your weight.

Apples

Apples can be part of a healthy diet that promotes weight loss because they satisfy hunger with only a few calories. A study at Florida State University showed that eating a cup of dried apples daily can help women lose weight and lower their cholesterol and heart disease markers. In addition, according to the *National Health and Nutrition Examination Survey,* diets high in dried fruits are associated with lower Body Mass Index (BMI) and improved diet quality.

Asparagus

Asparagus has an exceptionally high nutrient/calorie ratio and may be the perfect weight-loss food. Asparagus is a rich source of the soluble fiber inulin, which has been shown to suppress appetite. Asparagus is also a very low calorie food. In fact, asparagus is a negative calorie food, which means that more calories are burned digesting it than it provides. Asparagus also helps to maintain your blood sugar levels stable which can help you avoid crashes and binges that lead to overeating.

Avocados

If eaten moderately, avocados can play a role in weight loss diets. While they are high in calories, their high monounsaturated fat content helps to increase feelings of satiety. In addition, research suggests that exercise burns monounsaturated fat more efficiently than saturated fat.

Coconut

Extra virgin coconut oil can be a helpful tool in your weight loss efforts. It contains short and medium-chain fatty acids that help in taking off excessive weight. Coconut is easy to digest and it helps in healthy functioning of the thyroid and enzymes systems. It also helps to increase body metabolism and energy because it is more likely to be burned as fuel than stored as body fat.

Grapefruit

Research suggests that the chemical properties of grapefruit reduce insulin levels and encourage weight loss. Grapefruits have high amounts of fat burning enzymes, high water content, fiber and low glycemic load. A combination of these characteristics makes grapefruit a perfect food for losing weight.

Yogurt

Adding yogurt to your diet helps you lose weight by increasing your body's ability to burn fat, especially that stubborn belly fat. Your stored belly fat produces the hormone cortisol, which signals your body to store more body fat. The calcium in yogurt helps break this cycle by signaling your fat cells to produce less cortisol. The amino acids in yogurt also help you burn calories. According to a study published in the *International Journal of Obesity,* obese adults who ate three servings of fat-free yogurt daily as part of a lower-calorie diet lost 22% more weight and 61% more body fat than those who just cut calories. In addition, yogurt eaters also lost 81% more belly fat.

Wrinkles

As we age, the inner layer of the skin begins to thin. The skin begins to lose its stretchiness and structure. Although aging is inevitable, wrinkles don't have give your age away. The right foods can help you look as young as you feel.

Sweet Potatoes

The sweet potato's orange flesh color is directly correlated to its beta-carotene content. Sweet potatoes boast large amounts of this valuable nutrient which helps protect against UV damage and wrinkles.

Broccoli

Broccoli is high in antioxidants, including vitamins C and E which aid in the production of collagen, protects your skin cell membranes, guard against UV radiation damage, and keep your skin healthy and supple.

Papaya

Papayas are a great source of antioxidant vitamins C and E and carotenoids, nutrients which can help protect your skin against free radicals known to cause damage that leads to wrinkles and signs of aging.

CONCLUSION

Thank you for buying and reading this book. I sincerely hope that you found this book to be a valuable resource and that it has had a positive impact on you.

Best wishes!

Naya

ABOUT THE AUTHOR

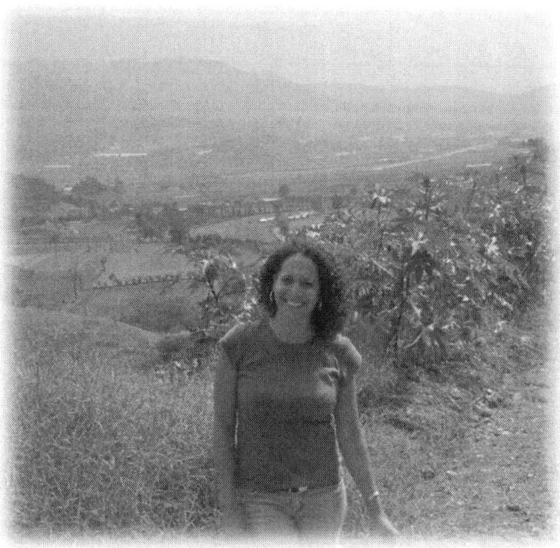

Naya has had a lifetime passion for natural and preventive medicine. She loves healthy foods (spicy foods even more), wine, and travel. She has lived in the Dominican Republic, Argentina and Taiwan. She now lives in the sunny state of Florida with her husband and family.

Naya is the author of:

HEALING FOODS: Practical Guide to the Health Benefits and Medicinal Properties of Food

REAL CLEVER SOLUTIONS AND IDEAS: Tips and Tricks to Help You Save Time and Money.

FREELANCE TRANSLATION HANDBOOK

Connect with Naya Lizardo

Twitter: http://Twitter.com/prioritytrans

Amazon Author Page: http://amzn.to/10T8oQD

4118589R00109

Printed in Great Britain
by Amazon.co.uk, Ltd.,
Marston Gate.